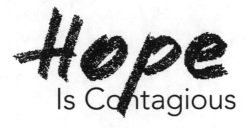

Hope
Is Contagious

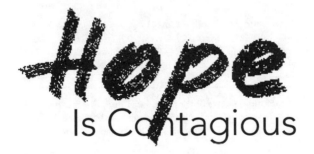

Hope
Is Contagious

DR. KEN HUTCHERSON

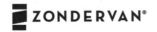

ZONDERVAN®

ZONDERVAN.com/
AUTHORTRACKER
follow your favorite authors

ZONDERVAN

Hope Is Contagious
Copyright © 2010 by Ken Hutcherson

This title is also available as a Zondervan ebook.
Visit www.zondervan.com/ebooks.

This title is also available in a Zondervan audio edition.
Visit www.zondervan.fm.

Requests for information should be addressed to:

Zondervan, *Grand Rapids, Michigan 49530*

Library of Congress Cataloging-in-Publication Data

Hutcherson, Ken.
     Hope is contagious : trusting God in the face of any obstacle / Ken
Hutcherson.
          p.   cm.
     ISBN 978-0-310-32768-4 (hardcover)
     1. Hope—Religious aspects—Christianity. 2. Trust in God.
3. Consolation. 4. Cancer—Patients—Religious life. I. Title.
BV4638.H88   2009
     248.8'6—dc22   2009046401

All Scripture quotations, unless otherwise indicated, are taken from the Holy
Bible, *New International Version®*, *NIV®*. Copyright © 1973, 1978, 1984 by Biblica,
Inc.™ Used by permission of Zondervan. All rights reserved worldwide.

Any Internet addresses (websites, blogs, etc.) and telephone numbers printed
in this book are offered as a resource. They are not intended in any way to be or
imply an endorsement by Zondervan, nor does Zondervan vouch for the content
of these sites and numbers for the life of this book.

Published in association with the literary agency of Wolgemuth & Associates, Inc.

Cover design: Extra Credit Projects
Interior design: Michelle Espinoza

Printed in the United States of America

10 11 12 13 14 15 16 • 20 19 18 17 16 15 14 13 12 11 10 9 8 7 6 5 4 3 2 1

*In the middle of all the cancer treatments and hospital runs
and my hectic day-to-day work and preaching schedule,
one man encouraged me to write this book,
and it is to him I dedicate it.*

To Dr. James and Shirley Dobson

*This book is dedicated to your lives and work
serving our Lord Jesus Christ.*

May you be richly blessed.

Contents

Acknowledgments

I f it takes a village to raise a child, it takes almost that many people to produce a book, and without them I could never have finished this project. I am grateful to my church, Antioch Bible Church in Redmond, Washington, for all of their support. They generously allowed me the time to write and gave me an opportunity to test-drive my ideas. I have preached on some of the themes in this book, and though my parishioners are always polite when I don't quite get it right, I knew when I had not really connected—and so I left that stuff out.

My assistant at the church, Rachael Whaley, has been my arms and legs as I wrote between trips to the hospital.

I am indebted to Dr. James Dobson, whose interview of me sparked interest in this book. If you'd like to hear this interview, visit *http://listen.family.org/daily/A000001976.cfm*.

My agent, Robert Wolgemuth of Wolgemuth and Associates, not only assisted with the business side of producing a book but also provided encouragement along the way. Robert also introduced me to Lyn Cryderman, who provided editorial and writing assistance.

I could not possibly thank everyone at Zondervan who took the manuscript and turned it into a book, but special thanks is due my publisher, Dudley Delffs, and my editor, Sandra VanderZicht. I will trust them to pass along my appreciation to everyone who marketed, publicized, sold, and shipped the book.

Introduction

What were they thinking?

When the producers of the movie *Letters to God* called and asked me to appear in their movie, I thought they must have had the wrong number. The name's Hutcherson, not Nicholson. I'm a preacher. On a good day, I might put on a pretty good show when I'm in front of my congregation on Sunday mornings trying to get an important point across, but no one would confuse me with Denzel Washington. True, I've been on film before — game films when in my other Sunday job I was a linebacker in the National Football League. But those game films hardly qualified me for an Oscar — except for the times I got flagged for roughing the quarterback and acted like it was an accident.

I loved hitting those little guys!

When I showed up for the filming of "my scene," I realized what was going on. They were just trying to be nice to this old guy. Here I was, all nervous about having to memorize my lines only to discover I *had* no lines! In fact, they were quite clear they didn't want me to say a word. "Just stand there, Hutch, and look concerned." Turns out they had heard my story and thought it would be nice to have me hang around the set for a few days. Of course I was thrilled because I knew this movie was based on a true story of how a boy who had cancer became an inspiration to everyone who knew him. In the movie and in the true story on which it was based, the doctors and medical people said little Tyler Doughtie had no hope.

Were they ever wrong!

Tyler's my kind of guy. Even at his tender age, he knew he had the most reliable hope known to mankind. He knew he was going to die, but that didn't stop him from trying to get the most out of life while he could. That's because he knew that playing soccer and hanging out on his little roof-top balcony with his friends was nothing compared to what was in store for him. Tyler must have paid attention to his preacher because he understood that when his life on earth was over, a better one awaited him. One without IVs and nausea. One where no one would make fun of him because he had gone bald from his chemotherapy treatments. A never-ending life in which he would be reunited with his dad and soon be joined by the rest of his family and friends.

When you have that kind of hope, you can face anything without letting it get you down. I've been a preacher now for thirty-two years, and I've seen how this hope not only sustains people going through tough times but attracts others to them, which in turn gives *them* hope as well. It's like a virus, and no level of protection can stop it from spreading. We can't help ourselves. When we see someone who has just been laid off yet who can still appreciate the beauty of a sunrise or marvel at a baby's smile, we're drawn to them. Sure, they're worried about putting food on the table, but they seem to have grabbed hold of something that's bigger than the challenge they're facing.

We're way too familiar with whining. We see it all the time, usually from people who appear to have everything they ever wanted. Nothing contagious about that. In fact, these are the kinds of people we try to avoid. You know what I'm talking about. They see a rainbow and complain about the rain. You never want to ask them how they're doing because they'll unload all their aches and pains on you. But think of all the people who've inspired you. I'm pretty sure they weren't the ones complaining about the weather or the economy or the Republicans or the Democrats. I don't know about you, but the people I like to hang out with are the ones who have been knocked off their horse and yet find a way to laugh about it.

What about you? What kind of person are you — better yet, what kind of person do you want to be?

I've been through a few tough times myself, and one time someone said to me, "I'm so impressed with your optimism in the face of all you're going through." Of course I thanked that person, but I had to correct them. "That's not optimism you're seeing," I began. "Optimism is something *I* do, and I'm just not strong enough sometimes to be optimistic. What you're seeing is hope, and that's not something I *do* but something I've been *given*."

If you saw me standing next to Tyler, you might come to the conclusion we have little in common, and you'd be right. He's little; I'm big. He's young; I'm old. He's white; I'm black. He's cute — OK, at least my wife thinks I'm pretty cute too. But both Tyler and I have something that no one can take away from us: *hope*. And we also know this isn't something we conjured up with our willpower or positive attitudes. It was given to us by God, who promised to let us live with him forever. When we have that kind of hope, nothing — absolutely nothing — can hold us down for very long. Hope like that changes the whole ball game because we already know the final score. Once we know we're going to win, we quit worrying about the game plan and just go out and get the most out of every day. That's what Tyler did, and it inspired his friends to do the same thing.

I'm writing this book because a lot of good people seem to be losing hope. Maybe you've noticed. You meet your buddies for coffee, and it's all gloom and doom. You listen to the news, and it seems as if nobody's doing anything right. I'm sort of tired of hearing everyone complain about how hard things are for them, aren't you?

I'll be the first to admit that times are tough and that a lot of scary things are happening in our world. But what could be scarier than learning you don't have much more time left on earth? Forget the economy. Forget unemployment. Forget rogue nations making bombs. I'm gonna die a lot sooner than I should! If a child can get that news and still have hope, you can too, and in this book I will show you how. I'll share some of my own story of how I went from being angry about my circumstances to being able to joke with the nurses in the emergency room, even though things were looking pretty bleak for me. I'll tell you some stories from the Bible that will point you toward that hope and explain why nothing bad can happen to a Christian. And I'll challenge you to tap into that same hope that Tyler Doughtie and I have—a hope that will not just help you survive but thrive, regardless of what life throws at you.

Fortunately, I got through my scene in the movie without too many takes. I'd like to think I'm a natural for the big screen, but to be honest, I just did what I was told and kept my mouth shut. I admit I was tempted to ad-lib a little in the hope that the director would "discover" me. I love being a preacher, but just think of all the good I could do for God if I were a movie star! Somehow he missed me, and you might too, unless you watch the movie very carefully. Here's a hint: my scene took place in the hospital.

What I don't want you to miss, though, is an opportunity to "catch" the true hope that is waiting for you. It's not a magic formula or a seven-step process but a gift that is offered to anyone who will accept it. Once you get it, you will wonder how you lived without it, because it will change everything. You'll still have your struggles, but they will no longer have the power to turn you into someone you don't want to be. And it won't just change you but everyone around you.

Imagine what our world would be like if a pandemic of hope broke out!

As I was putting the finishing touches on this book, a disturbing report hit the news about a little boy in Chicago who was shot and permanently disabled in a drive-by shooting. That fact alone is awful enough, but the reporter went on to say that everyone in the neighborhood knew who the shooter was, but no one would come forward to identify him. The boy's mother even acknowledged that she drove by the shooter's house every day on the way to work. But what caught my attention were the words of an educator from Chicago who was interviewed by the reporter. The quote went something like this: "That's what happens when people lose hope. You don't think things will get better, so you just give up."

I don't want to see *anyone* give up, especially when hope is so readily within our grasp. Whether you're walking the streets of the inner city of Chicago or sitting at your kitchen table, no tragedy can dim the hope that comes from knowing that God will walk with you through the valley and that his presence will give you peace because he is the baddest one in the valley. He held little Tyler's hand throughout his battle with cancer, and he will hold yours too.

Dr. Kenneth "Hutch" Hutcherson

October 2009

Don't Feel Sorry for Me

Seldom does someone have the chance to experience two life-changing events in one day. September 9, 2002, was my lucky day.

I was in Southern California for a meeting with John Wooden, one of the greatest men alive. His basketball teams won twelve NCAA national championships, something no other coach has ever done. ESPN named him the greatest coach of all time in any sport, and he has been awarded the Presidential Medal of Freedom, the highest civilian honor in our nation. This meeting gave me the opportunity—along with a pastor friend of mine, John Werhas; Los Angeles Lakers' coach Paul Westphal; Lakers' announcer Keith Erickson; and radio talk show host Larry Elder—to listen to and learn about life from John Wooden, clearly an American hero. What I always loved about Coach Wooden is that he was as concerned about the character and development of his players as human beings as he was about their basketball skills. I consider his seven-point creed one of the best guidelines to living anyone could ever find. It was given to him by his father when John graduated from grammar school:

1. Be true to yourself.
2. Make each day your masterpiece.
3. Help others.
4. Drink deeply from good books, especially the Bible.
5. Make friendship a fine art.
6. Build a shelter against a rainy day.
7. Pray for guidance and give thanks for blessings every day.

Not a bad guy to be around when someone is about to get the news I got before meeting him. Just before my friend John was to pick me up to go to Wooden's home, I got a phone call from my doctor. A few days earlier, he had discovered during a routine exam something that concerned him and had sent me to the hospital for a biopsy. I'm smart enough to know that doctors don't do biopsies for little stuff, and I gotta tell you — waiting for the results of that biopsy was tough.

So here I am, ready to head over to see one of my heroes, and the call comes in: "Hutch, the biopsy was positive. You have cancer."

As you'll learn later, I've been scared to death of cancer

all my life. I don't mean just a little worried that I might someday get the disease; I mean the kind of scared that wakes a person up in the middle of the night in a cold sweat. And I have to say, when I heard the news, it stopped me in my tracks. It totally took the wind out of my sails. But I was about to meet a guy I've respected all my adult life. Can't really go in there all worried about my own self. So I had to just suck it up and go out to meet Coach Wooden, and that was the best thing for a guy like me. It completely took my mind off the bad news I had just gotten and filled me with awe and wonder at such an inspirational guy. Most people are fortunate to experience one life-changing event in their entire lives. What are the chances of experiencing two such events on the same day?

I don't believe in chance.

While I wasn't exactly thrilled to learn I had cancer, being able to listen and learn from the great John Wooden made it a great day for me. For those ninety minutes or so, I forgot I had cancer and focused my attention on his practical wisdom and faith. He was well into his twilight years, but you wouldn't know it from his hopeful outlook. I was reminded we both shared the same hope that no matter what was going on in our lives, we had something better to look forward to. You can't help yourself when you're around people like that—their positive outlook just has to rub off on you.

Cancer? I think we're going to get along just fine.

I promise you I won't bore you with any of the details of my disease except for this. My form of cancer is confirmed in a test called the prostate-specific antigen (PSA) test. The results come in the form of numbers. A "score" of 0 to 4 is considered normal. If you score on a range from 5 to 7, the results are considered elevated and the situation must be closely monitored. Anything over 11 is a sure sign that something is seriously wrong. Over the last eight years, my PSA score has gone from 11 to 80 to 400 to 800 to 1,400 and eventually all the way to 1,800+. I'm a walking, living miracle because with scores this high I should be dead!

Over the years since receiving the news, I've been in and out of the hospital dozens of times. I've had to go to the emergency room so many times I should have frequent-flier status, or at least a room named after me. I've been in meetings where I've had to excuse myself so I could find a place to throw up, and then I'd have to go back into the meeting and try to concentrate on the work we were doing.

I used to be a professional football player — a linebacker — so I've always been a pretty big guy, and over the years since I left the game I've managed to stay in pretty good shape. But to look at me now, you'd think maybe I was one of those little placekickers. Except I'm black. We don't do field goals!

If you've ever ridden a roller coaster, you have an idea of what it's been like fighting this disease. Just when things start looking real bad, my doctors try another kind of treatment, and after dealing with all the side effects, I start to bounce back a little. I get some of my strength back. The pain—at least most of it—goes away, and I begin to feel almost normal again. For a while. Then it's back to worshiping at the porcelain throne. Not being able to sleep because of pain. Fatigue that feels like a lead blanket draped over my shoulders, weighing me down. And the knowledge that maybe this time I won't bounce back.

Are ya feeling sorry for me yet?

Well, please don't, because no matter how bumpy the ride, I'm enjoying it. Maybe not the pain and nausea, but the blessings that come from having to depend entirely on God and discovering that he's more than up to the task of turning this challenge into something beautiful. That's not just brave talk or the practice of "mind over matter." I'm not delusional either. I know how serious this thing is, and that my time here may be running out. I need to be really clear about this because I don't want to come off as someone who's trying to veil the truth because it makes a good story. If you knew me better, you would know I don't pull any punches. I tell it exactly like it is, even if it sometimes gets me in trouble (and it certainly has). So when I say I'm enjoying my trip with cancer, you can take it to the bank. I know it may not make sense to you right now, but it will. I've been living with this ruthless disease for seven years now, and the prognosis isn't good. I want to live as much as you do, and when it comes to pain, I hurt as much as anyone else. But I can say without hesitation that these years have been the best years of my life. Certainly not the easiest. Not the most pain free (by a long shot). But the absolute best.

Don't get me wrong. I certainly didn't ask for this cancer, and I would not object if God decided to heal me. I ask him to heal me every day and believe he could do it in a heartbeat. I'm not particularly fond of pain, and nausea has to be one of the worst things the human body ever dreamed up. But the truth is, I'm not just enduring this thing or *trying* to have a good attitude despite my disease. I'm having the best years of my life, and that's what this book is all about. Not cancer. Not healing. Not sickness. Not pain. Not death. But hope.

This book is about hope. Not a false hope that you'll never die, never suffer, never deal with disappointment or tragedy. If anybody tells you that you can go through life without ever being sick or being broken, they aren't telling the truth. What I'm talking about is a true, real, readily available hope that no matter what happens—no matter what circumstance you find yourself in—you can say with me, "This isn't nearly as bad as I thought it would be. In fact, it's pretty good." And mean it.

If you've ever thought, "I sure do hope that tomorrow will be a better day for me," this book is for you. If you ever hoped that you could be the person you always wanted to be, no matter what obstacle stood in your way, this book will show you how this desire can come true. If you're tired of the way things are in the world but think it's hopeless to bring about any changes, I think I'll be able to change your mind. But let me be real clear: I don't have a gimmick or a three-step plan for you. This isn't a self-help book; in fact, you may learn that one of the reasons life hasn't turned out the way you hoped it would is that you're trying too hard to help yourself.

I decided to write this book because I see so many good, decent citizens virtually overwhelmed by things over which they have little control. I'm writing this as the United States (and many other countries as well) is in the middle of a serious economic recession that seems to have put a dark cloud over everything. If you asked me to describe the mood of the country, I would use words such as *fear, despair, frustration,* and *cynicism*. Maybe even a little *anger*. The economy is just our current excuse for these negative emotions—emotions that have been around since the beginning of time and will be with us forever.

Anytime we let these feelings creep into our lives, it's deadly. I'm convinced that no one likes to stay in those dark places, but when I listen to people and watch how they live, it's as if they are caught in a whirlpool of negativism and can't swim their way out of it. What a shame, because regardless of the economy or our health or anything else that interrupts our world, we can still truly enjoy life! Rise above these circumstances, and enter a place of peace, joy, and contentment. You do not have to just hold on and try to survive — you can face whatever comes your way with courage and hope, finding dozens of reasons to smile each day, regardless of what's trying to drag you down.

In your heart, you know it's possible. Perhaps you've seen a friend or family member whose positive spirit in the face of hardship has inspired you. Or something planted deep in your soul tells you that your happiness should not be dependent on external circumstances. A friend of mine returned from a mission trip to Haiti, one of the poorest countries in the world. Like so many people who go on such trips, he went to minister to the poor and came away feeling as though the poor church folk had ministered to him. "They just had such joy, even though they lived in horrible conditions," he recalled. "And it was infectious because I found myself laughing and having a blast with my new friends, even though we were surrounded by such poverty."

Whatever you're dealing with right now, I'm pretty sure it isn't close to what a Haitian mom or dad is going through. I don't say that to make you feel guilty but to give you hope. If a Haitian mother living in a cardboard shelter can sing, with a radiant smile on her face, "The joy of the Lord is my strength," you can too. You can face anything in life — anything — and have that same inner peace and joy. And when you do, it's contagious. It lifts up everyone else around you. Isn't that the type of person you want to be? Instead of joining over and over again in the whining about how bad things are, just your presence shows others that, hey, life is still a wonderful gift we should all be enjoying.

I know what you're thinking: "This guy's a preacher, and he's going to lay some of that 'pie in the sky when you die' heaven stuff on me. No thanks."

It's true. I'm a preacher, and I believe in heaven *and* hell, and we'll talk about both because they have a lot to do with hope. I plan to spend the rest of eternity in heaven, and you might be there with me, but that's not doing much for either of us right now, is it? The hope that I'm going to share with you is for right here, right now. You don't have to wait until you get to heaven to escape the prison of disappointment and despair. I'm planning on celebrating forever in heaven, but I'm having a lot of fun right now, despite all those cancerous cells trying to kill me. You can too, regardless of what you're dealing with. I'll show you why no matter how hard you try to overcome the obstacles life throws in your path, they still get you down—and that they will always get you down, even if you try harder to overcome them. In fact, I'll tell you to *quit* trying. But I'll also show you how you can actually turn these obstacles into reasons for celebration. How the loss of a job or being stuck in a wheelchair or losing every penny of your 401(k) not only isn't as bad as you think it is; by the time we're done, you'll see that it is actually good!

The other day I was relaxing in my recliner after having spent five hours in the emergency room the night before.

I'll admit I was exhausted, and the pain medication wasn't working as well as I would have liked. I looked around and saw my family going about their lives as usual. Video games. Chores. Music. Laughter. My wife, Pat, was fixing breakfast. Even our new little puppy was settling into a comfortable routine and enjoying everyone's efforts to spoil him. A visitor stopped by to chat. Some friends from church surprised me with a birthday cake—I had almost forgotten it was my birthday. So there I sat, surrounded by so much goodness even as I'm feeling lousy. My favorite cake is staring at me, but I have no appetite. My eleven-year-old runs past me, and I don't have enough energy to grab him and wrestle him to the ground like I used to. I'm trying to have a conversation with my guests, but between the short night and the powerful pain pills, I can barely stay alert. And you know what I'm thinking? Can you imagine how close I am to being overwhelmed with what is happening to me?

The words practically shouted from inside of me: "Isn't God great? What a privilege to be his child!"

This book isn't about me. It isn't about cancer. I've only shared this much of my story to give you a glimpse into what *you* can expect. The life you always wanted—the kind of life in which at the end of the day, no matter what's going on in your life, you can say, "That was a good day."

Because it is. Even if things look bad. It's *all* good.

CHAPTER 2

What Are You Going to Do about God?

I grew up in a small town in Alabama during the 1960s, and like a lot of African-American teenagers at that time, I had a bit of a chip on my shoulder. OK, maybe a chip more the size of a boulder. It may be hard for you to believe this, but back then, we were actually taught that we black folks were only three-fifths human. Now what would *you* do if someone repeatedly told you that you were less than human? That you were 60 percent human (and who knows what they thought the other 40 percent was)? I decided early on that I would show those white folks. I would not just be as good as they were but better. I didn't aim for five-fifths; I was looking at *six*-fifths. Whatever I did, whether it was in the classroom or on the athletic field, I tried to be the best. I pushed myself like you wouldn't believe. In a way,

I'm grateful I grew up in that environment because it drove me to greater success than I might have had if I had been treated as an equal.

Being told I was less than human might also explain why I was such a terror on the football field. I loved all sports and lettered in football, basketball, baseball, and track, but football was my favorite because it was the one place where it was legal to hurt white people.

Trust me. Every chance I got on the football field, I flattened anyone who got in my way. Anyone. Black, white — it didn't matter, but if the guy was white, I'd drill him a little harder than usual. And sometimes, just for good measure, I'd nail one of the white kids as he walked back to the huddle after picking himself up off the grass from the first time I hit him. Oh, I was nasty! Of course, since I hit *everyone*, regardless of their color, the white kids never knew I was saving my best for them. Pretty sneaky, huh? It got so bad that my football coach wouldn't let me wear pads in practice to discourage me from hitting my teammates so hard. He needed everyone else to be healthy for the game on Friday night. Pads or no pads, I hit 'em anyway.

I was almost as wild off the field as I was on it. It's not that I got into a lot of trouble or messed with stuff I shouldn't be messin' with. Like I said, I aimed to be the best and had the discipline to stay away from anything that would make me look bad or get me into serious trouble.

Besides, I knew my grandmother would kill me if she caught me doing drugs or hanging out with thugs. I just lived life hard and fast. For example, I had a motorcycle, and one night I crashed it because I was driving way over the speed limit just for the sheer thrill of it. Very abruptly, however, the thrill was gone as I took a curve too fast, wiped out, and had to be rushed by ambulance to the emergency room at our local hospital. For the next five-and-a-half hours, the doctor and nurses scraped out as much dirt and gravel from my legs as they could and then stitched me back up. Before they started, someone said something about anesthesia, and I practically jumped out of the bed in protest.

"What's the problem, young man?" the doctor asked, clearly annoyed with me.

"I'm not lettin' any white man have at me while I'm sleepin'!"

"Son, you got a whole lot more guts than brains," he replied.

That's just the kind of kid I was back then. Angry. Distrustful. And a little on the wild side. The only religious influence I had was my dear old grandmother, but I wasn't much interested in church or the Bible. It seemed fine for the older folks in my town, but not for me. A tough guy like me didn't need *anyone* helping him, let alone someone you couldn't see. One time, however, I saw a movie that at least got me thinking about God. It was called *Angel Unaware* and starred Roy Rogers and Dale Evans. It was a pretty powerful story, but I remember thinking at the time, "I don't need you, God. I can make it on my own."

As far as I was concerned, my only chance of getting out of that little Alabama town would come from my own self. I didn't trust anyone to help me and I certainly didn't have any faith in a god who let white people treat me the way they did. Hope was what weak people did; it wasn't anything I needed because I was determined to make something of my life.

About a year later, we had an assembly at my high school featuring a speaker from an organization called Campus Crusade for Christ. Can you imagine that happening today at a public high school? I'll never forget the message from the speaker. He told a story about a guy named Boom Boom Bradley, who had a knack for making bad decisions at crucial moments in his life. I thought to myself, *Hmmm, that sure sounds like me.* I wanted so much to be better than anyone else, but it was becoming clear that I was my own worst enemy. When Boom Boom Bradley turned his life over to Christ, he started making better decisions. Hearing that story had a huge impact on me because no matter how hard I tried to do the right thing, I kept making stupid mistakes. I realized it was my own foolish pride that stood between me and God. I was too stubborn to admit I needed more than what I could do for myself, but the truth was, I wasn't doing so well with my self-improvement plan. So when the speaker gave an invitation, I was ready to accept what God seemed to be offering me. I remember thinking, "Here's God, Hutch. Whatcha gonna do with him?" I bowed my head and almost said out loud, "I'm yours."

I couldn't have known it at the time, but that decision ultimately gave me exactly what I wanted in life: the best.

First Step toward Hope

There are a lot of religious words to describe what I did when I bowed my head that day: *saved, converted, justification, salvation, invited Jesus in my heart, became a Christian.* The words don't really matter. What mattered is what happened in my heart, in the very depths of my soul. Some people make becoming a Christian complicated, but the Bible makes it pretty simple: "Believe in the Lord Jesus, and you will be saved." That's it. Do you believe Jesus is the Son of God? Then you're a Christian. Period. And now that you are a Christian, you have the ultimate hope. Hope for a better life here on earth, and hope for the best life forever in heaven. Nothing else the world offers can give you that kind of hope. Not money or fame or the right degree from the right university. In fact, over the years I've met a lot of people who have all those things and were still miserable until they surrendered their lives to God.

If you believe that Jesus is the Son of God, you have settled once and for all the most basic and important aspect of hope: you will live forever with God. That's not my opinion, but it's the truth. I recognize that in our "anything goes" culture, this statement may sound arrogant. We have been led to believe there is no such thing as absolute truth. So this may well be a good place for me to explain where I get my beliefs. How can I speak of "truth" with such certainty?

I was deeply influenced by my experience in team sports, so when I became a Christian, I transferred three important rules I learned from sports to my faith:

1. The coach is the coach.
2. You better know his playbook.
3. You do not change the plays.

God is in charge of our lives. Not us. Everything we need to know about how to live is in the Bible. Everything. And just because you run into something in the Bible you don't like, you can't change it, because *every word* of it was inspired by God and is true. When you start messin' with these truths, don't be surprised if things start to unravel in your life, because God's playbook was written for us so that we could be winners. God wants the absolute best for you, and if you follow his playbook you'll have the life you always wanted. You'll be a better parent, a better spouse, a better employee, a better citizen because God knows what you need to win at life, and he lays it out for you in his Word. For example, do you want to be a great parent? Don't provoke your children, cautions the Bible (Ephesians 6:4). Don't be afraid to discipline them (Proverbs 23:13). Teach them the difference between right and wrong (Deuteronomy 4:9). Introduce them to Jesus (Matthew 19:14). Follow this playbook for anything in your life, and you can't go wrong.

That may sound simplistic, but one of the reasons I'm able to rise above the pain and uncertainty of my cancer is that I follow that playbook to a T. The Bible tells me to rejoice in all things, so I find reasons to be joyful, no matter what. You ever hear someone laughing in the emergency room? I've done it many times, and it surely gets people's attention. Nothing funnier than a big black man like me trying to hold that hospital gown shut in back and walking with an IV cart at three in the morning! Pretty soon, everyone's laughing. Bone-tired doctors who've seen one patient too many. The tough guy who seconds ago was bragging about the bar fight that led to broken bones in his hand. Even the worried mom with a feverish and listless baby on her lap. Talk about contagious. All because I believe the Bible when it says to rejoice in all things. Do you think that instruction was put in there to play a joke on us or make us try to do something impossible? God knows that your attitude can turn a bad thing into a good thing, for yourself and for those around you. Not only did I feel better when I found a reason to laugh, but a whole bunch of people felt better too.

I remember one time when a nurse was trying to get an IV going on me. Only another cancer patient knows what that means—for the next several hours, medicine is going to drip into your body, and whether or not it kills the cancer, it's going to make you sick. Real sick. The kind of sick where at first you're afraid you're going to die, and then you're afraid you *won't* die. So I'm sitting there looking forward to *that*, and this poor nurse can't get the needle into a vein. She's poking away and getting all frustrated, and I'm thinking how funny this would be if I wasn't the pin cushion. Pretty soon she called another nurse to give it a try, and she couldn't get the needle into a vein either.

It eventually took three nurses working for an hour and a half before they got the IV in me, but I just talked to them the whole time, making jokes and apologizing for having such tough old veins. As the head nurse opened the valve that started the medicine drip, she thanked me for not getting angry, like most patients do when things don't go according to plan, and I responded by telling her I was just obeying orders: "God tells us to rejoice no matter what, and I figured he wanted me to do a lot of rejoicing; otherwise he wouldn't have let you jab me so many times." The nurses laughed so hard I briefly considered becoming a comedian.

God knows exactly what you need in order to experience the very best in life, regardless of your circumstances.

You Can't Earn Hope

You may have been led to believe that being a Christian means you have to follow this set of rules or that set of traditions, but the Bible doesn't teach this. This idea comes from denominations and other human institutions. The Bible never restricts people as much as denominations do. You don't have to join a particular church to be a Christian. You don't have to read the Bible every day. You don't have to quit smoking. You don't have to really *do* anything. In fact, the reason so many people have such a hard time being a Christian is that they think it's all about them. They think it's about being good. They think it's a list of rules. They knock themselves out trying to keep all those rules and then get mad when life throws them a curve. Shouldn't all that hard work and energy I expend trying to be good give me the hope I need to make it through the day?

Now to be fair, it is a good idea to become a part of a church that believes what the Bible says is true. Those who spend time reading the Bible will certainly grow deeper in their faith. And it's never a bad idea to give up *any* vice that's not good for you. But these things have nothing to do with your salvation. Nothing. You can't earn your way to God, because being a Christian is all about what God did, not what *you* do, and this is a big hint about hope. It's not just about what God *did* but about what he *is doing*. With or without you.

Real hope doesn't come from anything *you* do.

According to the Bible, you become a Christian by believing, and if you truly believe in Jesus, you will be a different person. The Bible makes it clear that salvation is *the* most important and necessary experience in your life that opens the door to hope. But it is a gift you receive, not a privilege you earn. You can be the best person in the world, but if you don't believe Jesus is the Son of God, you aren't a Christian. On the other hand, you can make a huge mess of your life, but if you truly believe Jesus is the Son of God, you're a Christian.

Two ice fishermen were standing beside a lake covered with ice. The first fisherman was sure the ice was thick enough to walk out on and go fishing. The second wasn't so sure. "Do you really believe it will hold us so we won't fall through?" he asked his friend. "Absolutely!" came the reply. "Then you go first." The first fisherman refused. Did he really believe the ice would hold him? Of course not, because if he had, he wouldn't have hesitated to march out onto it.

A lot of people who say they believe in Jesus are like that first fisherman. They say they believe he's the Son of God, but they don't do anything about it. Nothing in their lives has changed; therefore they don't really believe. The Bible says even the demons believe, "and shudder" (James 2:19). At least they know not to play games with God. *Saying* you believe and *actually* believing are not always the same thing.

When you put your faith in Jesus, you have been given the gift of eternal life with him in heaven. The Bible teaches that we will all live forever. Just think of that word for a moment. *Forever.* Consider the average life span of Americans — right around seventy-five years, a little longer for women. When you're a child, that amount of time seems like forever. When you are in your twenties, you're not even thinking about that thing called retirement because it seems so far away. But talk to someone who's approaching even fifty or sixty years of age. They always say something like, "My, the years went by so fast," or, "It seems like just yesterday I was graduating from high school."

Eternity began before people walked the earth and will continue forever after we die. Compared to eternity, the few years we spend in this life are like a dot on a piece of paper stretching to the farthest planet and back. Are you sure you want to live that "dot" the way *you* want to instead of the way God wants you to live?

I've often said that if every human being could spend just twenty-four hours in hell, everyone would be a Christian. The Bible teaches that hell is a place of eternal suffering. That bothers some people, and even some preachers and theologians ignore this biblical teaching or try to explain it away. "It's just a metaphor," they say. "God would never make anyone suffer like that."

What if they're wrong? Are you really willing to take that chance? When you pick and choose what parts of the Bible you believe, those are the risks you face. With what's at stake, doesn't it make more sense to buy the whole package? (I'll talk more about heaven and hell in chapter 9.)

If you have confessed your belief in Jesus as the Son of God, you have the glorious hope of living with him in heaven forever and the promise of God's presence to comfort and encourage you in your journey here on earth. If you haven't yet decided what to do about Jesus, what's stopping you?

Great Expectations

Here's what often happens when a person becomes a Christian. They get all fired up about reading the Bible and growing in their faith. They see with clearer vision the evil that surrounds them and often join worthy causes to fight for truth and righteousness. They are so overjoyed about what happened to them that they want to share it with others — to introduce them to the same new life they received. Then after a while they get discouraged because the causes they join don't seem to be making much impact. The "bad guys" almost flaunt their ungodliness while the "good guys" get mocked on late-night television. When these sorts of things happen to Christians, they often begin questioning God. Then something bad happens to them. It always does. The plant where they've worked for eighteen years shuts down; their marriage hits a huge bump in the road. And then they begin to wonder, "If God really cares about me, why did he let this happen to me? If he's in charge, why is our world in such a mess?"

Do you remember the *Saturday Night Live* skits featuring

Dana Carvey as "the Church Lady"? Even though these sketches were intended to mock religious people, they were pretty funny. I recall one skit where someone complained to the Church Lady about the way Santa Claus shifted the focus of Christmas away from the birth of Jesus. Church Lady agreed that this was a terrible thing, and then, rearranging the letters of Santa's name, she raised this now-trademark question, "Could it be—SATAN?"

Well, actually, despite the sarcasm of this skit, the Church Lady was theologically correct. The Bible teaches that there is a force of evil at work in the world, and therefore life can never be perfect. But this fact doesn't mean we just give up and let evil run free in our world. It's good to stand up for what's right—I do it all the time. I'd like to tell you that if we all just tried harder, we could create a perfect world, but I wouldn't be telling you the truth. I'd love to hold out hope that someday, in our lifetime, we'll completely eradicate bad things such as abortion and pornography; greedy CEOs and crooked politicians. But again, I'd be lying—offering false hope. I take a stand for God primarily out of obedience. He hasn't given up entirely on the world and expects us to do everything we can to make it a better place. But it will never be perfect. Not yet, anyway.

I'd also like to tell you that if you just put your trust in God . . .

you'll never lose your job.

you'll always have enough money to pay your bills.
no one in your family will get sick.
your friends will never let you down.
your kids will never disappoint you.
no one will ever wrongly accuse you.
your spouse will never leave you for someone else.
your boss will never make your life miserable.
you will never face a serious tragedy.

Who wouldn't want to promise you these blessings — and many preachers do! But the truth is, you can love God with all your heart, keep his commandments, and devote your entire life to serving him, and you can still lose your job.

Not to brag, but I've pretty much sold out completely to God. I *live* everything I write about in this book. I've taken a lot of hits as I stand up for things that honor his Word. I've been loyal to my wife and family. I obeyed his call to become a preacher, I don't hit white people anymore, and I've made the Bible my handbook for living, believing every single word contained within it. And guess what?

I'm dying of cancer.

Some of you have been unable to accept the Christian faith because you cannot accept a "good and loving God" who would allow a guy like me to suffer from an incurable disease. OK, I understand you may not care much about me, but you've had a family member who did all the right things for God yet lost her life to a terminal illness. And some of you have accepted Jesus but struggle with your faith because you think it's unfair that someone who believes in Jesus and lives according to his teachings gets laid off while the guy next door who lives for the Devil keeps climbing the corporate ladder. Both of you have one thing in common: you are looking at your situations from *your* perspective instead of God's. And you are looking at life from a temporal or short-term perspective rather than an eternal one.

I Want It My Way

If you're a parent, have you ever experienced one of your children insisting on doing something his way when you knew "his way" would be harmful to him? For example, you live on a busy street. There's a neighbor kid your son likes to play with, but he lives in a house across the street. Your little five-year-old runs toward the street because it makes sense to him that to play with his friend he needs to get to his friend's house. But you know that what makes sense to him can get him killed or badly injured. So you grab him and tell him he can't cross the street unless you go with him and hold his hand. If no one's looking, you might even give him a little smack on the behind for emphasis. He might argue. He might throw a tantrum. He might try to pull his hand out of yours and cross the street anyway. But you hold your ground. You don't much care whether he likes your way or not, because you are smarter than he is and more interested in his safety than his happiness.

From your son's point of view, you seem stern. Unfair. Bossy. He may think you're trying to prevent him from enjoying his life. That you're trying to make him miserable just because you're bigger. If he was older, he would probably call you "repressive." You probably don't relish these regular power struggles with your child, but you know it's part of being a good parent. He's concerned only with what is right in front of him — a chance to play with his friend across the street. You have a much longer view of his life and want to help shape it to be the very best life possible.

Or how about when you must discipline your child? You see behavior that if allowed to continue will either harm him or lead to the development of poor character. For example, you expect your teenaged son to make his bed and keep his room clean. It's not that you're a neat freak or like to flaunt your authority. Instead, you know that the discipline of keeping his room clean molds him into someone who is industrious and well organized. You also know that holding him to a standard prepares him to be a good employee and productive citizen. If his room starts to get messy and, even after a few warnings, his bed remains unmade and his clothes are strewn all over the floor, you decide to ground him for a weekend. *He* thinks you're being mean and that you don't love him, but *you* know it's out of your love for him that you are trying to shape him into becoming a better person.

Isn't it funny how this makes sense to us when we think of our children, but when God allows something to happen to us that we don't like, we start acting like our own kids. We question him. We argue with him. We rebel against him. If you are a good parent, you don't let your children's arguments against you change your behavior. It would be irresponsible and very likely cause even greater harm for your child. Unfortunately, especially as our children approach their teen years, many parents let their desire to be liked overrule their commitment to love their children, and then they wonder why their teenagers get involved in harmful and often dangerous behaviors.

God is a good parent, but first and foremost he is God. Theologians use a term to describe him in relationship to mankind: *sovereign*. It's a term usually ascribed to governments; it simply means the person or persons in power have the undisputed right to make decisions. In a monarchy, the king or queen has unlimited and absolute power. That's sovereignty. My football coach was a great coach, and he expected us to treat him as if he was sovereign. But he was fallible. He could make mistakes. God is perfect. He cannot make mistakes. If I obeyed my coach, who could and sometimes did call the wrong play, why would I *not* obey God, who is *incapable* of making a mistake?

Here's another key to understanding hope: Only when we put our complete trust in the sovereign God can we experience true hope. Tyler Doughtie lived fearlessly and joyfully, even though he had an incurable disease, because of his simple trust that God had everything under control.

When I made the decision to believe in Jesus, I went after it like I did just about everything else. I went right home and began studying the Bible like I was going to take a test. Imagine being a senior in high school and studying the Bible five hours a day — sometimes more. That's what I did, because I decided that if I was going to be a Christian, I was going to be the best. That's when I made the commitment that I would never compromise on anything that was in the Bible. It was my playbook, and I wasn't going to change it, even if at times I didn't like or fully understand what I was reading.

I still gave 110 percent in the classroom and on the football field. I knew I couldn't afford to go to college, so football became my hope for a degree — and it worked. Despite a lot of college coaches' concerns about my motorcycle injury, I was given a scholarship to play football at the University of West Alabama and hit enough people hard enough to get noticed by the Dallas Cowboys organization, which drafted me. I loved playing in the NFL, but all the money and adulation you get as a professional athlete didn't mean very much to me because I knew my *real* calling. God had made it very clear to me that he wanted me to serve him as a preacher, so when an injury ended my career, I wasn't overly upset because it meant I could get going on what God wanted me to do.

The human side of me would like to take credit for the intensity with which I pursued my faith, but this trait is a gift from God. Remember, he's sovereign. In control. For whatever reason, he instilled in me this hunger for his Word and a single-minded commitment to follow him whatever the cost. But despite my deep faith and obedience, I knew there was something holding me back. Even as a child, I had this overwhelming fear of cancer. I'm not exactly sure why, but it doesn't matter. In many ways you might have described me as fearless, especially if you watched me play football. But deep inside, I was scared to death of cancer. I couldn't imagine anything worse than being told I had it.

Now let me ask you something. If you were sovereign — all-knowing, all-loving, and all-powerful — if you had undisputed power to mold a person into whom you wanted him to be, why would you allow him to face the thing he is most afraid of? Why would you take someone who was so single-minded about serving you and give him a disease that not only made him suffer but limited the time he would have on earth serving you, the sovereign one?

Think about it, as we take a look at how God dealt with a spoiled brat.

High Hopes for a Lowly Slave

I'm not sure why I had such an intense fear of cancer, but for as long as I can remember, I thought it was about the worst thing that could happen to me. It seemed as if once a person was told he had cancer, it wasn't long before he was gone, and the process of going wasn't very pretty. In God's perfect timing, he gave me that meeting with Coach Wooden right after my diagnosis because he knew I would have been a complete wreck if I didn't have something as inspiring as that experience to distract me from the news. Let me tell you, after being with this great coach, you couldn't help but be pumped up about life, which is probably why I left that meeting ready to fight.

Whatever it took, I was going to beat that disease right out of my body. I started to feel like I did when I was in the NFL and the oddsmakers picked us to lose. It just brought something out in me that made me want to prove them wrong. I didn't doubt the doctor's *diagnosis*, but I wasn't about to accept his *prognosis*. Cancer became that crosstown rival that came into my house and scored a big touchdown and was now strutting around in the end zone, certain of victory. Not so fast, chump. The Hutch is gonna smack you down big-time!

When I finally got back home, I told my wife. We decided to wait until we could all be together for dinner before I told our children. I was still in the fight mode and tried to put a brave face on things as I shared the news: "My doctor told me today that I have cancer," I began. As you might expect, they were stunned. Normally, family dinner time is pretty noisy as we get caught up on each other's lives while we grab for another piece of my wife's fried chicken or meat loaf. But all of a sudden it got real quiet. I could see the concern in their faces and naturally wanted to calm their fears, even as I was scared silly inside. "But don't worry. I'm gonna fight it and beat it. Together we'll get through this." Although I had tried not to show it, the seriousness of my situation sunk in when my daughter Avery blurted out, "Are you gonna die, Daddy?" Leave it to kids to get right to the point!

"I'm not planning on it, baby," I answered, but cracks had already started to form in my resolve. Just hearing her ask that question brought all my fear bubbling to the surface. I knew that they were watching me, though, and that my countenance would dictate how my entire family would deal with this news. So I sucked it up, answered a few more questions, and then began eating a dinner for which I had absolutely no appetite. Business as usual. They saw that I wasn't overly shook up about it and planned to beat it, and apparently that was enough for them. "Game on," as they say.

Over the next few weeks, however, fighting it wasn't working. Despite my bravado, inside I was falling apart. The more I fought my cancer, the more frightened I became. I would research the disease and study the different treatments, but the only thing that seemed to accomplish was to make me realize just how serious it was. I began to think about something none of us think about much — that I might not be around much longer. I have to admit, it hurt. I wasn't at all worried about my final destination, but what about my family? I hated the thought of leaving my wife to care for our children on her own, and thinking about my kids being without their daddy was nearly too much to bear. So I focused all my energy on getting rid of this awful disease. I prayed earnestly for God to heal me, but I also told my doctor I wanted him to unleash every medicine and therapy at his disposal to zap those enemy cancer cells. But no matter how hard I tried to fight it, I kept spiraling deeper into fear and depression.

This went on for about a year until I felt like I just couldn't go on anymore, and that's when God reached out and grabbed me. I was exhausted from the effects of my cancer and all the drugs inside of me uniting to fight it, and I was just plain tired of being afraid. And that's when it sunk in. During my entire ministry, I had taught people about God's sovereignty and how he has everything in control, but here I was trying to handle this challenge by myself. Sure, I prayed about it and let God know how I was feeling, but deep down inside, this had become *my* battle. I had given him everything else but had kept this one thing for myself. It was almost as if God had been waiting patiently in the wings until I couldn't fight anymore and then he put his arm on my shoulder and said, "OK, Hutch—you ready to let *me* handle this now?" I had made cancer my enemy, but God wanted me to allow him to use it to teach me more about him.

Beware of that one thing in your life you want to hold on to, because one way or the other, God's going to get hold of it.

From that point on, I made cancer my pastor. Instead of fighting it, I would learn from it. Each trip to the emergency room in the middle of the night would become a sermon teaching me yet another lesson about God. Instead of viewing my disease as an accident, I would recognize it as something God allowed to happen so that I could learn to love and trust him more than I ever had. I had always taught that God allows us to suffer so that we can become more like his Son, Jesus—now it was time for me to live what I preached.

Once I decided to let my cancer teach me more about

what really matters in life, God began to introduce me to others who have let cancer become their pastor—a person such as Paul, a man who has liver cancer. He needs a liver transplant that will cost $1 million and follow-up medical care that totals around $50,000 a year. And he doesn't have any insurance. We talk on the phone almost every week, and you know what he always says? "God's in complete control of this thing. Whatever he decides to do is going to be the absolute best thing for me."

Then there's my "girlfriend," Gerry. She and I were diagnosed around the same time and have been living with our cancer for eight years. Gerry is eighty years old and loves the Lord with all her heart. I've actually seen her praise God when she's gotten bad news. As I write this, Gerry just received the last of her current round of treatments. If these treatments prove ineffective, the doctors give her three to six months. You think that's got her down? No way! She's an inspiration to all the people at the clinic who care for her—and to me as well. I figure if an eighty-year-old woman can trust God no matter what, so can I.

Some people have a problem with the idea that God will put hardships in our way to accomplish his purposes, but the Bible makes it clear that he will do whatever he has to in order to build his kingdom. Just think of all the heroes of the Bible whom God allowed to suffer for his sake. If you grew up in church and went to Sunday school, you probably heard the story of Joseph at least once a year. And just as many times you probably used crayons or construction paper to create your own design of his "coat of many colors." The story is so popular that I'm convinced if you asked a perfect stranger on the street who wore that coat of many colors, you'd get the right answer.

Most people love this story because of its happy ending, but I like it because it shows what it took to get Joseph to that ending. For us to have the kind of hope that allows us to face anything and still be joyful and content, we have to understand sovereignty. Joseph's story is a good place to start.

Dad Loves Me the Best

I know that most people think of Joseph as a great man, but in reality he started out as a spoiled brat. It wasn't really his fault. Kids don't spoil themselves—their parents do the spoiling. You really can't blame Joseph for being the last child of his father, Jacob (also known as Israel). Talk to any older brother or sister about their youngest sibling and they will generally proclaim that this child had it a lot better than they did. And apparently Jacob did not have a great deal of instruction in parenting because the Bible tells us he "loved Joseph more than any of his other sons" (Genesis 37:3). And just to make sure the rest of his sons knew that, Jacob made a "richly ornamented robe" for him. Not exactly the best way to endear Joseph to his older brothers. Where I come from, the younger you are in the family pecking order, the more raggedy the hand-me-downs. But Joseph got a brand-new jacket.

Can you imagine what it must have been like for those brothers?

"Hey, Dad, where's *my* robe?"

"Sorry, Issachar, you don't get one."

"Why not?"

"Because I don't love you as much as I love Joseph."

And can you imagine what it must have been like for Joseph? He didn't ask to be favored by his father, nor did he ask for a robe made of the finest linens of various colors with diamonds and gold and other precious stones woven into the fabric. Then again, he could have hung it up in his closet and saved it for special occasions, but instead he wore it around the house for all of his brothers to see. Just the sight of their privileged punk brother must have been difficult to deal with. It was like wearing a sign to remind them where they stood in their father's eyes. According to the Bible, they didn't deal with it very well: "they hated him and could not speak a kind word to him" (Genesis 37:4).

Talk about sibling rivalry!

It didn't help much that Joseph also had this quirky habit of sharing his strange dreams with his brothers. I mean, your dad lets everyone know he loves you more than all the brothers, you're strutting around in your fancy jacket, and then you call those brothers around you and tell them your dream:

"Hey, guys, I had this dream, ya know, where we were, um, out gathering grain, and my bundle of grain, like, stood tall and proud while your bundles of grain bowed down to mine. Gee, I wonder what *that* means."

His brothers didn't wonder. They knew Joseph was trying to tell them he would some day rule over them, and it just made them resent him even more. You'd think Joseph would get the message and maybe tone it down a little, but he went to them with yet another dream:

"You guys won't believe this dream I had last night. This time, the sun and moon and eleven stars were bowing down to me. Go figure."

Hmmmm, let's see. Joseph had a mother and a father and eleven brothers. It didn't take a rocket scientist to get what Joseph was saying: "Not only will all of you guys bow down to me, but Mom and Dad will too!" You may not think of him as spoiled, but at the least he lacked any sense of how his special status offended his brothers. The Bible says that this dream only made them more jealous of their spoiled little brother, and it turned out to be the last straw because the next chapter of this story finds the brothers plotting to kill him. Joseph travels to a nearby village where his brothers are tending the flocks. They grab him, steal his jacket, and throw him into a cistern.

I'm guessing this was a major wake-up call to Joseph. He thinks he's all that with his fancy robe and spared the hard work of tending his father's flock. That dirty, dusty manual labor was work more suited to his brothers. He's being groomed for management. He gets to go check on them and report back to his father — and suddenly he's in a dark and deep hole in the ground, and his treasured robe is gone. Where I come from, we call that cutting him down to size. Teaching him a little humility. Only these guys were out for blood. It wasn't enough to humble Joseph; they wanted to kill him. One of the brothers, Reuben, convinces them to spare his life, so they sell him to some traveling merchants, who take him to Egypt and sell him to one of Pharaoh's officials, Potiphar.

One day you're the apple of your father's eye; the next day you're a twice-sold slave. One day I'm preaching and building up my church and enjoying my family; the next day they tell me I have cancer. A little boy is minding his own business growing up, and then he finds himself in the hospital with an IV in his arm. It's just not fair, right?

Here's where it gets interesting, so pay attention. Joseph could have folded his cards and become just another sullen, angry slave. He could have whined to God about the unfairness of his situation. Instead, he rose above his circumstances and became an awesome servant. Honest, diligent, hardworking. The kind of slave that makes whatever you paid for him a bargain. So Potiphar put him in charge of his entire household, trusting him to take care of everything he owned. If you had to be a slave, this was about as good as it gets. He had the run of the place and apparently could do no wrong because the Bible says "the LORD blessed the household of the Egyptian because of Joseph" (Genesis 39:5).

What happens next is a warning for anyone who achieves a level of success. Right when Joseph is at the top of his game, Potiphar's wife tries to seduce him. Even as I write this, I'm reminded of at least two prominent politicians—both professed Christians—who recently were forced to confess they were unfaithful to their wives. Both men were at the peak of their promising careers—some believed both had a shot at running for president some day. Of course, the press thinks it's all about sex, but it's not a sex thing at all. It's a sovereign thing. When things are going great for us, we begin to think we're in control. We can do anything, and no one is going to ever find out. Power, success, achievement, fame, wealth—they all delude us into thinking *we're* sovereign. And when we make ourselves sovereign, we lose hope.

That's why at first I was so scared about my disease. You see, I made it *all about me.* Even though I had preached so often about sovereignty, I held on to this one area of my life, making it my battle and doing my best to defeat this enemy. My only hope was myself, and relying on myself wasn't working because I was consumed with fear. What kind of hope is that? God wants *every* area of our lives. He can't be 99 percent sovereign—he is either in complete control of everything or has no control at all.

Joseph knew all about sovereignty. We learn from the Bible that he loved God, and when the beautiful wife of his master asked him to go to bed with her, he honored God by refusing, saying, "How then could I do such a wicked thing and sin against God?" (Genesis 39:9).

You would think this would be a good place for the story to end. Joseph takes a big stand for God; God rewards him for his obedience with a beautiful young woman who falls in love with him. They get married, ride off into the sunset on a white horse, and the curtain falls on a great moral tale: Do what's right, and God will give you all that you desire.

Not exactly.

God is not all that interested in giving you everything you want. Instead, he wants to give you his best. Big difference!

Thanks a Lot, God!

Potiphar's wife is livid with Joseph and decides to turn the tables on him. She runs to her husband and claims that Joseph tried to rape her. Potiphar responds by throwing Joseph into prison. I don't know about you, but facing a trumped-up rape charge after you just took a stand for God's righteousness would make me wonder if God really knew what he was doing. Maybe this sovereign stuff isn't all it's cracked up to be.

A lot of us might crawl over to the corner of our cell

and curse our foolishness for not buying what Potiphar's wife was selling. Forget this God thing. I could have had some fun, and I'd still be large and in charge. But Joseph apparently did not let this new turn of events get him down. We learn he was such a model prisoner that the warden put him in charge of the entire prison. He looks after a couple of prisoners who were once on Pharaoh's staff, and as they are released, he must be hoping they'll put a good word in for him so he can get out soon. Again, here is a good place for the story to end. Unfairly accused felon sticks with God's program and gets an early release. Instead, one of the Pharaoh staffers loses his life (in fulfillment of Joseph's dream interpretation), and the other staffer forgets all about Joseph — and so Joseph spends another two years in prison.

Finally Joseph is released. Pharaoh had begun to have some odd dreams and can't find anyone to interpret them, but the guy from his staff who had been in prison with Joseph finally comes through and recalls this amazing young Hebrew man who seemed to be a dream expert. So Joseph is summoned, and he interprets Pharaoh's dream. Pharaoh, of course, is so impressed that he puts him in charge of his entire palace and declares, "All my people are to submit to your orders" (Genesis 41:40). Joseph implements his famous famine relief plan, which saves the Egyptians as well as the Hebrew children of God from perishing. When he is finally reunited with his brothers, who fear he will take revenge on them for what they had done to him, he puts in perspective his entire life and all the suffering he experienced: "Do not be angry with yourselves for selling me here, because it was to save lives that God sent me ahead of you.... So then, it was not you who sent me here, but God" (Genesis 45:5, 8).

Do you realize what he was declaring in that state-ment? This is our playbook. The Bible. God's word to us — in my opinion, absolute truth you can entrust your life to. And here's the truth that Joseph's life is saying to us: "God orchestrated *all* the events that led to his saving his cho-sen people. He allowed my father to spoil me so that my brothers would hate me so that they would ambush me and put me in an abandoned well. He empowered Reuben to save my life so that I would be sold as a slave to one of the closest advisers of Pharaoh, the ruler of an empire that could easily have eliminated the entire Jewish population. He tempted me with a beautiful woman who was married to my master, and when I chose righteousness over evil, he had me thrown in prison — not as punishment but to put me in an even more influential position with the Egyptian government so that I could be an instrument to save the children of Israel."

Now let me ask you something. Do you believe God is sovereign? Do you believe he knows what he is doing and has the authority to do whatever he wants or needs to do so that his kingdom triumphs over evil?

Joseph believed it. I've got to believe there were times he was discouraged. An earthen well and a dingy prison cell are not very pleasant places, and he must have questioned whether or not his God had his best interests in mind. He took a huge hit for spurning the advances of a beautiful woman—don't you think he had a few second thoughts as he was carted off to prison? There's nothing wrong with questioning God, but at the end of the day, Joseph decided to trust God—no matter what. To believe that whatever happened to him was part of a bigger plan that had eternal implications not only for him but for the entire kingdom of God.

Now here's the coolest part of this story. When the dust finally settled and Pharaoh realized that Joseph had reconciled with his brothers, he said this to Joseph: "Tell your brothers, 'Do this: Load your animals and return to the land of Canaan, and bring your father and your families back to me. I will give you the best of the land of Egypt and you can enjoy the fat of the land'" (Genesis 45:17–18).

Over his relatively short life, Joseph dealt with several things that from a human perspective were totally unfair and made his life miserable. Who would have blamed him if after his brothers sold him he just caved and turned his back on God? Or when he was in prison on the rape charge and a couple of government officials asked him to interpret their dreams, no one would think ill of him if he just told them to get lost and then served his time the best he could. Instead, he trusted God—even when it seemed as if God had abandoned him—and not only was the nation of Israel saved; they were given the *best*!

Get Yourself Out of the Way

One of the strange things about the human condition is that the more we focus on ourselves, the more miserable we become. I got so wrapped up in fighting cancer that I couldn't see what God wanted to do for me. I've come up with a little acronym to describe people who make life all about themselves: MESI — miserable, exasperating, stinking individuals. You see them everywhere. Married people who want to get out of their marriage because "my needs aren't being met." Workers who grumble because "the other guy got the promotion." Children who have their iPods, designer clothes, flat-screen TVs in their bedrooms hooked up to their Wii systems — and they're bored! The more you get your way, the less you enjoy your life.

This isn't about possessions, though. It's about *position*. About where you stand in relationship to God. If *you* are the most important thing in your life, you are always going to be a MESI. I guarantee it. You may occasionally enjoy periods of happiness or pleasure, but overall you will be unsettled and unsatisfied. Restless. Worried. You will feel as if the life you had always hoped for is just out of reach, and you'll make yourself even more miserable trying to attain it. And when things happen to you that you don't like, you'll go into a tailspin. Life's not fair. God must not care about me. What did I do to deserve this? But after your little pity party, do you feel any better?

On the other hand, if you give God his rightful place

in your life and trust that he's in complete control, you begin to see the things that happen to you in a new light. It's almost as if you have to get yourself out of the way so you can see God and know that he's got everything under control. When my doctor called me to tell me I had cancer, all I could think about was *me* and how *I* was going to fight it. Fight it — big-time! I was the bad boy linebacker again, and cancer was that running back coming at me. I made it adversarial. But the more I fought it, the more fearful I became. I wasn't winning, and I didn't like it. My entire focus was on what *I* was going to do about it, and that approach was making me miserable.

Yet the moment I recognized that, despite the cancer, God was still in control, I began enjoying life again. My fear was replaced with hope. Even if it didn't feel like it, I reminded myself what I had always believed: God knows what he is doing. His ways are *always* right. He is incapable of making a mistake. So I quit fighting. Instead of an adversary, this condition became a gift. I know this may be difficult to believe, and it's not like I *want* to keep the cancer. I still seek the best medical treatment I can find, and I pray to God that I will be healed. But my joy in life is not dependent on whether or not God chooses to heal me. I am able to live with my cancer and enjoy the ride because I *know* that God is sovereign. Whatever he chooses to do is good, so this has to be good.

Several times in the biblical account of Joseph, we see

these words: "the LORD was with him." When he was sold as a slave, "the LORD was with Joseph" (Genesis 39:2). When he was thrown in prison on false charges, "the LORD was with him" (Genesis 39:21). Whenever bad things happened to him, it was as if God was right there beside him saying, "I'm here. I know you can't possibly understand why this is happening, but just keep remembering who I am. I know what I'm doing, and I've chosen you to do it with me." What could be better than knowing that God is with you, no matter what's going on in your life? In my painful times, I have been almost overwhelmed with the knowledge that God is right there by my side. Where else could you possibly want to be than with God?

In the previous chapter, I asked you to consider why a sovereign God would allow someone who served him so well to suffer calamity. What could possibly be gained by letting someone who loves God so much experience hardships?

I'm convinced that when Joseph's brothers jumped him and threw him in a well, he had no idea what was going on. He couldn't see the "big picture." But he knew there was one. And he knew that God was the artist. That was enough for him. Why was he able to carry on and give his very best? Why didn't he try to escape and come back and kill his brothers? What gave him any hope of some day getting out of prison?

Sovereignty.

That's really the difference between hope and

hopelessness. Everything in our lives hinges on believing in God's sovereignty. God is God. You either accept it or reject it; there's no in between. You don't accept his sovereignty when things are going great and then reject it when bad things happen. If you reject it, you're on your own. Are you really willing to trust yourself when tragedy strikes?

If you accept God's sovereignty, you know that nothing bad can happen to you. You might be thrown into a cistern. You might be sold into slavery. You might be stuck in prison, forgotten by all. But it's all good. Your life doesn't fall apart. You might actually be able to sing and dance and enjoy yourself. Because no matter what, it's all good; it is part of God's unique plan for you.

When I first started going to the clinic for my treatments, I was scared to death. I tried not to show it, but deep down inside I felt like Joseph at the bottom of the well, and the light at the top of the hole kept getting dimmer. Now when I show up at the clinic, I'm the guy who lights up the place. All the nurses and doctors seem happy to see me, and I *know* it's not because I'm so good-looking. And even though I know they're going to shoot me up with poison that tries to kill more bad cells than good ones, I actually look forward to these visits because every smile and wave and high five reminds me that God has me right where he wants me.

Can you think of a better place to be?

Why Good People Do Bad Things

I f you've hung with me this far, you know that the hope I'm talking about comes from your relationship with Jesus. One of the reasons Tyler Doughtie, in the movie *Letters to God*, could face his disease with such a great attitude is that he had not only accepted Jesus as his Savior but also lived for him every day. With his simple, trusting faith he was such an inspiration to others because he reflected the very image of Christ in all that he did. When another kid made fun of him, he resisted the temptation to strike back and actually prayed for him. His letters revealed a heart for God and a desire to share his faith with all of his friends.

Sadly, a lot of Christians struggle so much to live the way God wants them to that they miss out on the blessings he has for them. It's like they can't quite be the people they want to be. To put it another way, why would anyone want what you've got if it looks exactly like what they have too?

You might have the hope that comes from knowing you'll spend eternity with God, but what good is it doing for you right now if you're just as miserable and mixed-up as your neighbor? The truth is, a lot of Christians are.

A friend of mine grew up in a little town in the Midwest where he attended a typical country church. As a youngster he attended Sunday school and sat through seemingly never-ending sermons about heaven and hell. Like a lot of children across America in the 1960s, he responded to the simple call of the gospel by asking Jesus into his heart.

"My Sunday school teacher told us that if we had Jesus in our hearts, we would go to heaven when we died, and we would live forever with God and our moms and dads," my friend recalled. "It just made sense, so when she asked us if we wanted to invite Jesus into our hearts, I said, 'Sure!'"

As my friend entered his adolescent years, he encountered all the things an adolescent boy encounters. "Once I was in the town's only drugstore with my friends, and they all grabbed candy bars and hid them in their pockets, so I filched one too," he remembered. "I felt so bad about it that I actually took it back after my buddies went home."

He continued to struggle with life's little temptations into his teenage years. Here's how he put it: "I don't know if the things I was tempted to do were sins or not, but based on how I was raised, I knew they were wrong. My parents didn't smoke and taught me it was wrong, so of course when one of my buddies produced a pack of cigarettes, we went behind his garage and tried it out. Another time, one of my buddies somehow got his hands on a torn and wrinkled copy of a magazine called *Photoplay*, which basically was a collection of pictures of women in skimpy bathing suits. Whenever we did stuff like that, even though I enjoyed it at the time, I always felt guilty afterward. I would go to my church's youth group and hear the talks about living the Christian life, and it would strengthen my resolve to not give in to all these little temptations. But the next time one of the guys would suggest something like sneaking some beer out of his dad's refrigerator, I'd go right along with the gang."

Sound familiar?

For the most part, Christians want to do the right thing. I don't know of anyone who wakes up in the morning and thinks, "Today I'm going to cheat on my spouse," or, "I'm going get drunk and drive my car tonight." On the contrary, most of us begin each day expecting to do our work well, treat others properly, and enjoy life's simple pleasures. So why, then, do Christians cheat on their spouses, drive under the influence, get angry over little things, lie to cover up their mistakes, gossip about others over coffee, or do any number of things that make life miserable for them and others?

Or to put it another way, why can't we be like little Tyler Doughtie and reflect Jesus in the way we live our everyday lives?

If you've read the New Testament, you have probably heard about the apostle Paul — one of the great saints of the church. A courageous missionary, Paul traveled throughout the entire Mediterranean region proclaiming the gospel to people who had never heard it before. Another of Jesus' followers, Luke, describes some of these expeditions in the New Testament book of Acts — literally an account of the "actions of the apostles" or followers of Jesus. For Christians, this book may be one of the most exciting and encouraging books in the Bible because it describes how a movement that began with Jesus and his twelve disciples spread like a virus. Paul's story is remarkable in that initially he was notorious for his persecution (read killing) of Christians. But once God got hold of him, he couldn't stop preaching, even after it landed him in prison. Over and over we read that the church grew in large numbers after Paul preached.

From super-sinner to super-Christian — that's our man Paul. So wouldn't you expect that a guy like this had it all together and never got tripped up by life's temptations? Move ahead to the New Testament book of Romans, where Paul meticulously explains his beliefs about the Christian faith and then makes this confession:

> I do not understand what I do. For what I want to do I do not do, but what I hate I do. . . . I have the desire to do what is good, but I cannot carry it out. . . .
>
> When I want to do good, evil is right there with

me. For in my inner being I delight in God's law; but I see another law at work in the members of my body, waging war against the law of my mind and making me a prisoner of the law of sin at work within my members. What a wretched man I am!

Romans 7:15, 18, 21–24

Chili Con Carne Christians

How can someone as spiritual as Saint Paul struggle with right and wrong? Isn't being a Christian all about doing the right thing? Yes and no. Do you remember how in chapter 2 we learned that being a Christian isn't about what you do but about what God has already done? Going to church every Sunday doesn't make you a Christian. Giving all your money to the church doesn't make you a Christian. Even obeying God's call to be a preacher doesn't make you a Christian. Being a Christian has to do with your *position* before God. Before you confessed your belief in Jesus, you were alienated or separated from God. Outside of his family. Once you confess your belief that his Son is the Savior of all mankind, you are joined with him. Part of his kingdom. Where before you occupied a position of guilt, now you are guilt free. And because of that, you will be with God forever.

Accepting Jesus as your Savior can be compared to a murderer having his death sentence commuted. You were guilty and deserved the sentence, but God generously pronounced you "not guilty," opened the doors of death row, and let you go. You're no longer guilty, but you aren't really free either. Your salvation gave you the wonderful gift of eternal life with God, but it didn't eliminate a condition that you have lived with and that has always made your life less than what it could have been—namely, your carnal nature.

If the word *carnal* is unfamiliar to you, think of its root as found in the title of one of my favorite dishes: chili con carne, or "chili with meat." Or more accurately, "chili with flesh." Throw a little cow in my chili, and I'm a happy man.

Your carnal nature is essentially that side of you that is governed by your flesh, or your earthly desires—sex, food, money, and other pleasures. You know what I'm talking about. There's nothing intrinsically wrong with these desires. God gave them to you. But if they are the driving force in your life, they will ultimately destroy you. Thankfully, you have another side to you—your spiritual nature.

Your spiritual nature is that part of you that desires to be the perfect person God originally created. It's the side of you that sees a homeless person holding out a little paper cup and asking for some spare change, and your heart is filled with compassion. It's the side of you that reports on the IRS tax form 1040 every penny you earned not because you are afraid you will get caught but because you want to be a person of integrity. On a good day, our spiritual nature wins out, while on a bad day that old carnal nature seems to rule over us like a tyrant. Most days they just fight with each other.

Some people teach that it is only after we become Christians that we have a dual nature — that before we accepted Christ we only had a carnal nature. But this isn't true, according to the Bible. Earlier in Romans, Paul explains that even those who are not Christians possess a spiritual nature. We call it "the conscience," and it is what moves people who do not know or honor God to still obey his laws.

Before I gave my life to Christ, I knew the difference between right and wrong. I remember one time I considered peeking at another student's paper during an exam. Just thinking about doing it made my heart beat so loud and fast that I was sure the teacher would look up and catch me, so I kept my eyes at home. That pounding in my chest was my conscience or spiritual nature. The very fact that I knew I had to sneak a peek instead of just blatantly look over at another student's paper is proof that I knew it was wrong, which proved I had a spiritual nature. God had written on my heart his commandment against stealing. People who have never heard of the commandment against stealing or who were never raised in a home that taught it was wrong to cheat would still feel that conscience knocking at their heart's door because God has created all of us with a spiritual nature.

Most people are able to let their conscience help them

do the right thing most of the time. But even the most morally upright people eventually lose the battle with their carnal nature. When this defeat occurs, we're usually surprised. We say, "He was such a good guy; I can't believe he would do something like that." But being a "good guy" on your own isn't enough. Eventually you will do something that you know is wrong—something you didn't really want to do but did it anyway.

Several years ago, a highly respected Christian leader confessed to an extramarital affair. This guy was one of those people who just seemed to have such a close walk with God that when the news became public, everyone responded with disbelief, then with great sadness. With everything he had going for him—a wonderful wife and loving family, the respect of the Christian community, several bestselling books about living the Christian life—how could he have let his guard down? Thankfully, he humbled himself before his family and friends, submitted to accountability with a small group of pastors, and restored his relationship with God and his family. But some twenty-five years after this confession took place, he told a group of men at a men's retreat, "Even at my age and after what I've been through, I'm still tempted when I see a beautiful woman." This time around, though, his spiritual nature controls him.

Sadly, many Christians continue to lose the battles between their spiritual and carnal natures. The major difference between them and those who are not Christians is that when Christians struggle, they feel horrible about it because they truly want to please God. When an unbeliever gives in to his carnal nature, he might be disappointed in himself, but it's not the end of the world for him. It's that sovereignty thing again. In essence, he is his own god. He let himself down, and he will just try harder the next time or simply accept the fact that "this is how I am." The Christian, on the other hand, knows that he deliberately disobeyed God. He knows that the conscience that urged him not to do something was his spiritual nature—essentially the Spirit of God—telling him to stop. The unbeliever is violating his own personal moral code, while the believer is sinning against God. Big difference!

Hopelessly Repulsive

Whenever a Christian struggles unsuccessfully with his or her dual nature, the damage moves in two directions—inwardly and outwardly. Back in the day, some of the old saints of the church would greet each other by asking, "Have you got the victory?" It was a sort of homespun accountability, reminding each other that the Christian life ought to be filled with the joy and contentment that come when we live right. Regardless of your circumstances, you could be at peace because you had victory over sin.

When you allow your carnal nature to control you, the initial damage is to yourself. You miss out on the abundant life God intended you to enjoy. The reason so many

Christians are conflicted about their faith is that they are carnal Christians, living in Romans 7. They have settled the question of where they will spend eternity, but they are making their own lives a living hell. They have resigned themselves to believing this is as good as it gets, but their spiritual nature tells them they could be enjoying a much better life.

Carnal Christians are often joyless, complaining, and covetous individuals. They are seldom happy because they keep looking at their circumstances from their own perspective, not God's. So when something bad happens to them, they complain because they think life is treating them unfairly. They always seem to be looking at others, wishing they could have someone else's job or home or car or marriage because theirs isn't good enough.

In addition to making their own lives miserable, carnal Christians hurt the church. They give unbelieving people a false image of the Christian life. Can you blame people who have developed critical and even antagonistic attitudes about Christianity? Contrary to a major misconception, it is not our positions on moral issues that cause people outside the church to disrespect us; it's our inability to live in a way that is consistent with what we say we believe. Our critics call it hypocrisy, and it comes from letting our carnal natures have dominion over us. We talk a lot about joy, peace, and contentment, but live like everyone else. Nothing contagious about that!

Imagine working in an office next to a woman who

is always cranky, critical, and complaining. One day, she arrives late to work because of car trouble, and the rest of the day she bad-mouths her husband for not keeping it well maintained. Your boss springs for ice cream for everyone in the department, and she mutters that she'd rather get the extra money in her paycheck. Over the months you learn that her kids are a pain in the neck, her neighbors don't speak English ("Why do they even come here?"), the cruise she took with her husband was a disaster, and her tennis club increased her membership fee. Then one day she comes up to you, all sweetness and nice, and invites you to a special event at her church. Do you think you would want to go anywhere near that church?

As a pastor, I have the wonderful opportunity of working with people who are earnest about God. The vast majority of the people who attend our church have settled the question of belief and participate in the life of the church because they want to become the people God wants them to be. They want the best for themselves, their families, and their neighbors and have learned how to thrive, no matter what's going on. Nothing pleases me more than to see people enjoying their lives, regardless of their circumstances. Trust me, our people face everything from unemployment to chronic illness to wayward children to foreclosure, and you seldom hear them complain. It's not because of me but because they have decided to trust God's sovereignty and believe the truth contained in the Bible.

Bury Your Sinful Nature

Even though being a Christian is not about what we do but what we believe, this fact doesn't mean that a Christian should continue doing things he or she knows are bad. Not only is your sin displeasing to God; it's making you miserable. The hope of eternal life that you received when you turned your life over to God is a priceless gift, but the Christian life also promises hope for the here and now. You don't *have* to always feel as if you don't measure up, nor do you have to allow the normal mishaps that occur in life to get you down, and here's where it begins to get exciting. You really *can* live a life that is controlled by the very Spirit of God, and it's not about trying harder.

When the apostle Paul wrote his letter to the saints in Rome, he knew he was writing primarily to members of the Jewish community who had become Christians. The Jewish people were (and still are) good people who loved God and tried to live according to the laws of the Old Testament. Not just the laws we call "the Ten Commandments." I'm talking hundreds of laws that governed every aspect of life. Laws about what you could and couldn't eat. Laws about what kind of clothes you wore. Laws describing the types of animals suitable for sacrificing as an offering to God, as well as precisely how they were to be prepared for the sacrifice. There are even laws in the Old Testament about mildew! To be a good Jewish person, you were required to follow all of these laws to the letter.

When members of the Jewish community in Rome converted to Christianity, many continued to obey the laws they had been taught since they were children. That, in itself, wasn't a big problem. For example, many of the dietary laws were designed by God to promote better health, and there is certainly nothing wrong with a Jewish Christian eating food that the Old Testament laws prescribed, even if it means he's missing out on a big plate of ribs. However, some of the leaders of these new Christians in Rome were teaching that following these laws was a requirement for remaining in the family of God—that their "goodness" (the Bible uses the term *righteousness*) depended on how closely they followed the Old Testament laws.

Paul knew that if they kept trying to be good by obeying the old laws, they would never fully experience the blessings of the Christian life. He explained that when Jesus, according to God's grand plan, died on the cross and then rose from the dead, the power of sin was broken, freeing us from having to live by the old laws. In fact, in Romans 3:20, Paul explained that "no one will be declared righteous in [God's] sight by observing the law."

In other words, quit trying so hard and start enjoying your new life!

If you're frustrated about the constant and unsuccessful struggle between your spiritual nature and your carnal nature, this should be great news. According to the Bible, when you accepted the gift of God's salvation, your old carnal self was defeated so that you could enjoy a new life, one that is "set free from sin" (Romans 6:18). Instead of continually trying and failing to live the life we know God wants us to live, we can relax in the knowledge that this good life we desire is already ours. To put it in the simplest of terms, before we accepted God's salvation, we were "bad"; when God saved us, he made us "good." It's a done deal. It's as if he is saying to us, "OK, I've made you a good person, so go out and act like one."

Does this mean you will never sin again once you believe in Jesus? Of course not. We're still human, and there is no such thing as a perfect human — with the exception of Jesus, who took on human flesh and lived on this earth for thirty-three years.

"But wait a minute, Hutch. Didn't you say earlier that sin was defeated? Aren't you just playing word games with me?"

When Jesus was crucified, he took your sins to the cross, and they were buried with him in the tomb. As such, they lost their power to control you. Sadly, sin is still present in the world and will be until Jesus returns to establish his eternal kingdom. But in the meantime — as in right now — you are considered by God to be righteous, or good, and the inability to stop doing bad things no longer describes you. In your past life, you were helpless. But now you have a powerful ally in the Holy Spirit — the very Spirit of God — who warns you when the temptation to do something wrong comes your way and who gives you the power to resist. God gives you the resources to live a life that is pleasing to him — and thus a life you will thoroughly enjoy. Those resources weren't available to you before; you were completely on your own. Rather than just try harder — which will never work — your responsibility is to listen to the Spirit and receive his power.

Practically Speaking

In the real world, here's how it works. Here's how you can put your head on the pillow every night with a clear conscience, knowing that sin has lost its power over you. First, you need to understand that, since you have become a new person in Christ, you are the one who chooses to feed your carnal nature to sin. Because of the Holy Spirit, you can't just sin off the cuff. It is impossible to just accidentally slip into adultery or casually fall into an angry spirit. You have to feed that impulse, deliberately cutting yourself off from the power you have been given over sin. In other words, now that you have a new life, you've got to *want* to sin. It's got to be a deliberate choice for you.

If you are a married man and a beautiful woman moves in next door, you're going to notice her. You're human. But even as you notice her, the Holy Spirit is going to whisper in your ear, "Watch yourself, big guy." If you're smart, you'll listen. You won't feed that carnal nature by hanging out in the backyard when she takes a dip in the pool. If you do, you'll hear the Spirit raise his voice a little: "Hey! Wake up! Quit feeding that old nature of yours, or you're going to get yourself in a big mess." In other words, you don't have to fight this thing alone. If you keep listening to the Spirit, he will remind you of the wonderful family he gave you. He will lift your thoughts toward him and away from whatever is tempting you. If you listen to the Spirit, you will be tapping into his power, which gives you the strength to resist the temptation.

As you feed your spiritual nature, you protect yourself from the power of sin to make you do things you really don't want to do. Using the example above, feeding your spiritual nature means the minute you notice that other woman's beauty, you will go to your wife and tell her she's gorgeous. Give her a hug—and maybe invite her to go out for ice cream. When you do that, you are feeding that spirit inside you that loves your wife and wants to enjoy a happy life with her for as long as you live. Feeding your spiritual nature means you will develop close friendships with a couple of godly men and tell them what's going on so they can slap you upside the head with some honesty and accountability. Feeding your spiritual nature means spending time each day praying and listening to God because all he wants for you is the very best, and if you pay attention, he'll give it to you.

When you think of these two natures, think of the old Eskimo who had two fighting dogs, a black one and a white one. He would take his dogs into town every week and unleash them to fight, taking bets from other men as to which one would win. Somehow he always won the bets. Someone once asked him how he knew which one would win, and he replied, "Whichever one I feed the week before I come to town. The dog I don't feed is going to lose because he has no strength."

If you want your spiritual nature to win, you have to feed it. You can't get around it. I don't care how spiritual you pretend to be or how good you try to be. If you don't feed your spiritual life, the carnal life will win and dictate what you do. In another New Testament book, the letter to the Philippians, Paul gets real practical as he describes how we can feed our spiritual natures: "whatever is true, whatever is noble, whatever is right, whatever is pure, whatever is lovely, whatever is admirable — if anything is excellent or praiseworthy — think about such things" (Philippians 4:8).

Notice that Paul doesn't say you have to *be* true and noble and pure. You just need to *think about* these things. Make them your mind-set. Immerse yourself in all the wonder and glory of life. How easy is that? One of the reasons I'm able to rise above the pain and uncertainty of my disease is that I purposefully focus on the good that surrounds me. I may be too tired to join in the fun, but being in the living room as my kids run in and out of the house is one of those "whatever is lovely" moments for me. And what could be more "excellent or praiseworthy" than experiencing the expert care and unwavering devotion of my wife? Friends stop by to cheer me up, and I know for a fact that most of the five thousand people at my church pray for me every day (the ones who don't will begin to after they read this!). And you know what else? I love to preach, and despite my cancer, God has somehow given me the strength to be able to keep preaching — except for one Sunday when I just couldn't summon the strength to do it. All these years of fighting cancer and only missing one Sunday! These are the things I think about, especially when I get another bit of bad news. Imagine the impact if every morning you took a few minutes to think about all the good that surrounds you.

When you let your mind wander around the landscape of excellence, there's little room for your carnal nature to intrude.

The more you feed your spiritual nature, the less likely you will give in to temptation. But as I said earlier, you're not perfect. You will make mistakes. Even with the Holy Spirit warning you and offering his power to protect you from sinning, you will sin. But here's the wonderful difference between a carnal-controlled Christian and a Spirit-controlled Christian. When you allowed your carnal nature to control you, each time you failed to live up to God's design for your life, you forgot about God's sovereignty. You looked at yourself through your own eyes and considered yourself a failure instead of looking at yourself as God sees you: his beautiful child who he has made righteous. You willingly returned to a position of guilt rather than grace—and likely beat yourself up a bit along the way: "I'm just too weak; I'll never be the Christian I want to be."

The Spirit-controlled Christian knows that God is sovereign. Sin may rear its ugly head occasionally, but it has been defeated. So instead of wallowing in shame and guilt, the Spirit-controlled Christian immediately confesses her sin to God, asks for his forgiveness, and moves on. She neither begs for forgiveness nor accepts it lightly, knowing that, though it is freely given, this forgiveness required Jesus' death and resurrection to make it available. But in that simple act of confession, she has freed herself from the power of sin to control her.

I heard a story recently about two close friends who both loved the Lord. They had one of those relationships that could be accurately described as "brothers in Christ." Devoted husbands and fathers and active in their churches, they met often for coffee before work. It seems that one of the men had developed an attraction to Internet pornography. It was one of those things that began out of curiosity but developed into a habit. After a few months of clicking into inappropriate websites, his conscience (spiritual nature) got the best of him, and he confessed this addiction to his wife and to his friend and resolved to stay away from raunchy websites.

He did all the right things to keep this sinister vice out of his life. He gave his wife his password and asked her to periodically log on to his computer and check his "footprints"; he set his computer so that it would filter out adult websites; he asked his friend to hold him accountable by regularly asking him about his Internet habits. I know this is a hard habit to break, but apparently this man was able to keep this area of his life pure. Yet, despite his success, he was burdened with such shame and guilt that, as he confided to his friend, he still felt distant from God.

After several weeks of listening to the guy whine about his past behavior and how lousy he felt about himself, his friend grew impatient. "I'm really tired of hearing how bad you feel about what you did," he began. "Don't you believe that Jesus died on the cross to save you from that sin?"

"Of course I do," he replied.

"Well, then, start acting like it! Jesus paid the price for your sin so that you don't have to."

Life as a Christian is not without temptation. And since Christians are human beings, life as a Christian is not without sin. You can continue as a Christian to let sin control you, to exercise its power to prevent you from having the life you truly desire. Or you can enjoy the abundant, joyful, and guilt-free life God wants you to enjoy. It's all about sovereignty. You either let God be God, or you keep trying to help him out by fighting your battles all by yourself.

I am convinced that most people really do want to live honorable lives. They inherently know — both from their own consciences and from human history — that the carnal temptations that promise pleasure and excitement never deliver anything but disappointment and shame. That the moral shortcuts we take because it seems easier only make things worse. If you are growing tired of trying to be good, maybe you should quit trying and start believing. God has won the victory over sin, which means you don't have to let it control you. The hope you have as a Christian isn't just for an eternal life in heaven but for a godly life on earth as well.

It's this kind of hope that draws the hopeless toward us, so that we can share its source with them.

Do you believe it? Start acting like it.

How Can Something Bad Be Good?

When I'm up in front of my people preaching and I say things they love to hear, the church gets a little noisy. People shout out "Amen!" or "Preach it!" when I remind them that God wants to give them the absolute best in life. You might expect that in a black church, but we're a kaleidoscope of all races and colors, and it's not just the black folks who shout. You wouldn't dare call our lighter-skinned people "God's frozen chosen" if you saw them getting excited when I get to preaching about heaven. When I tell them how much God loves them, they nod their heads and smile and throw out a "Praise God." When I remind them that God has a purpose for them, it gets a little louder and you might even see a few people standing up and moving a little. But when I start talking about *how* God achieves his purpose for them, it gets real quiet.

When I preach about Romans 7—the verses in which Paul agonizes over his inability to do what he wants to do—they get it. They know what it's like to try so hard to live decent lives, only to fail over and over again. I've never really had anyone question the whole teaching about the sinful nature and spiritual nature we all have. Even people who are not Christians understand the struggle over doing what's right. And when I move into Romans 8, which begins with the great news that there is now "no condemnation for those who are in Christ Jesus," the whole place erupts with gladness and thanksgiving. It's the news they want to hear, and they begin to realize they don't have to try so hard. God gave them Jesus and thus settled the question of salvation. They know their position before Christ, and it's good. God also gave them his Spirit to warn them of trouble and give them the power to stay out of trouble. It's their escape from the roller coaster of trying and failing, trying and failing—and that's good.

But then I have to tell them the rest of the story—the part of God's perfect story that most of us have such a hard time with: You can avoid eternal punishment by receiving Christ as your Savior; you can overcome the power of sin to control your life. But you can't avoid suffering. Not only can you not avoid it, but God allows it to happen to you. And that's good too.

Ouch!

You're serving God with a clean heart. With the Holy

Spirit's help you've conquered your old habits that kept you from being the woman he designed you to be. Where it used to be a struggle to go to church regularly, you're there when the doors open. You've even volunteered to help with the youth group—now there's a saint if I've ever seen one! Then on Monday, you learn that you didn't get that job you applied for.

Ouch!

Or you've been a real trooper for God over the long haul. For twenty-five years you have faithfully given more than 10 percent of your paycheck to the church. You run the church's food pantry, personally delivering food to homeless shelters. You still hold hands with your wife when you go out and have been a faithful and loving husband to her. The two of you are true pillars of the church. Then one day your wife is on the way to work, and a drunk driver crosses the center line and crashes head on into her car and her life is snuffed out.

Ouch!

Now here's the double ouch. When you come to me in your sorrow, I will hurt with you, cry with you, grieve with you. As a pastor, one of my greatest privileges is to be present with my people when they are going through the valley. So when you are heartbroken over the loss of your wife, I'll be there. And I will assure you that God is still in control. That he knows how badly you hurt and he is right there with you. And when you ask me why God would allow something like that to happen to your beloved wife, I will tell you the truth: "because he loves you."

Are you still with me? Can I get an amen?

No Part-time God

If you want to have the contagious hope that allows you to face any difficulty and triumph over it, you have to understand this biblical principle: There is no such thing as a bad circumstance in the life of a Christian. I was scared to death of getting cancer, and then when I got it, I thought something bad had happened. It took a year of fighting it before I saw that even when it came to cancer, God had a purpose for me. Once I understood this, it changed my entire outlook on my illness—so much so that I went out and got a vanity license plate: "No Fear." And it's true. I'm not afraid of anything or anyone, and it's all because of what I learned about God's sovereignty.

I know that this question of why God allows suffering has troubled people for ages—both those who believe in and trust God and those who don't. Many people have gone to great lengths to try to explain it on *their* terms. The atheist, in fact, uses this question to rationalize his inability to believe in God: How could a loving God allow the people he supposedly created to suffer? They simply cannot believe in an all-powerful God who would not use his power to prevent suffering, and therefore they conclude he doesn't exist.

Many Christians also cannot accept the fact that God

could allow suffering, so they try to solve this dilemma by saying that there are some things that are out of his control. That because a kind and loving God couldn't possibly want someone to suffer, those bad things must happen in spite of him. They just happen. In essence, they are saying that God only works part-time. That he's working in your life when he blesses you with a job or good health, but when you lost your job or got sick, he was taking a break.

Still others try to explain the problem of suffering by saying that God put his "natural laws" in place and then sits back and lets nature run its course. Because of gravity, if you fall off a cliff, you're going to eventually hit bottom and either die or get seriously injured. You just fall like a rock. God can't do anything about it because he would be violating his own laws. He invented gravity, which is a good thing, except when you stumble off a cliff. These people believe that God has the spiritual side of life covered and is actively involved with those things, but when it comes to sickness, accidents, money, relationships, and the like, you're on your own.

To varying degrees, those and other ways of trying to explain why bad things happen to those who love and honor Christ make sense when we look at life from *our* perspective. But they make no sense at all if you look at life from *God's* perspective, which he makes very clear in the Bible. Not to beat a dead horse, but it's that sovereign thing again. Either God is God, or he's not. He is either sovereign — in complete control — or he's not. Nothing is outside of his control, nor does he ever take time off. He is God all of the time, and everything he does is good — even the things that seem bad to us.

This might be a good place to remind you that this is a book about hope. Not hope for a better life, but for the best life. Hope that replaces fear with confidence, despair with courage. None of the above explanations offer hope. They basically tell us that bad things are going to happen to you, so deal with it. God may come alongside to comfort you in your time of trouble — which is true — but that's about all you can hope for. Just grit your teeth and bear it.

Hope like that is nothing but a Band-Aid.

Trust me, as one who has been comforted many times by God when I have been sick, it is a wonderful blessing to know we are never alone in times of need. Maybe you've experienced this too. In your darkest hour, when it seems as if everyone else has abandoned you, the very presence of God by your side is so real that you know you are not alone. It is the only thing that keeps you going. I don't want to minimize this blessing that all believers have, but there's more. Remember, God wants you to have the best.

Shortly after Paul shares with the Jewish Christians in Rome the liberating truth that they are no longer slaves to guilt and have the power to live victorious lives, he apparently anticipates the disappointment and discouragement they might experience the moment something bad happens to them, despite this new life. He knew that many of these new Christians would face horrible persecution; that many would even be killed because of their faith. He could have told them that God loves them so much that he would never let anything bad happen to them. That because they had committed their lives to Jesus they would always prosper. What do you think those believers would have done when the rocks started flying and some of their friends or family were thrown to the lions? "So much for this 'no condemnation' thing. Life wasn't all that great before, but at least no one was trying to kill me."

Paul probably knew what they wanted to hear, but he had to tell them the truth. And if you believe God is sovereign and his word is true, then what Paul has to say about suffering is worth paying attention to. For if we can grasp this important truth, it changes everything about how we face everyday life.

So Paul explains that when you become a Christian, you become one of his children. Since you are his child, you are also one of his heirs. As an heir, you get to share everything with Christ, including his suffering. Why? I mean, I can understand God sharing Christ's compassion and mercy with us. And I'm absolutely thrilled that he shares Christ's victory over death with us so that we can live with him forever.

But why his suffering? " ... in order that we may also share in his glory" (Romans 8:17).

Glory is kind of a funny word, isn't it? A little old-fashioned maybe. I'll bet you haven't heard that word used by any of your friends lately. Even if you have, it's not the sort of word we use to motivate people, so you might not be overly impressed with Paul's explanation of why Christians suffer. "Let me get this straight, God. I get to go to my child's funeral today so that I can get some glory?" Back in the day, one of the old sisters in church would get so excited about something the preacher said that she would raise a hand to the heavens and shout, "Glory!" To be honest, it was a little embarrassing. So if you're thinking "glory" isn't such a great trade-off for your suffering, I don't blame you.

If we drill down a bit on this idea of glory as a reward for our suffering, it starts to make more sense. The most common meaning of the word *glory* is "praise." So at the very least, Paul is saying that you will be praised or admired for your suffering. Back in my football-playing days, it was not unusual for a teammate to get injured in a game. Sometimes seriously. Whenever that happened, the rest of the team would run over to the injured teammate and lay some praise on him. If you were the injured player, you knew how much your teammates admired and appreciated you, and while it didn't take away the pain, it made it seem less important. I never, ever wanted to get hurt on the field, but when it happened, it was almost like a badge of courage. Have you ever heard the phrase "No guts, no glory"? It means you have to pay the price to get the praise. So Paul is telling us that our suffering won't go unnoticed.

Now this may seem like small consolation, however, until you consider *what kind* of glory our suffering produces: *his* glory, *Christ's* glory. In other words, the misfortunes you face give you the opportunity to experience exactly the same glory or praiseworthiness that Jesus received. It's one thing to get a pat on the back from someone at church when you're going through hard times. I'll admit I love it when someone from my church comes up to me and says something nice about the way I'm dealing with this cancer thing. But that's nothing compared to being able to share in Christ's glory.

Now here's the icing on the cake. The word *glory* also means "to make radiantly beautiful." That's what happens to us when we go through the fire. I love the final chorus of Handel's magnificent oratorio *Messiah*—"Worthy Is the Lamb That Was Slain." The words of the chorus come, appropriately, from the final book in the Bible, the book of Revelation. It acknowledges that Jesus was crucified so that *we* could receive "power, and riches, and wisdom, and strength, and honor, and glory, and blessing." That's what the cross does for us.

And then the chorus resounds with this tribute to Jesus: "Blessing and honor, glory and power be unto him." Are you with me? You and I as mere mortals are allowed to suffer so that we can receive the identical glory that the Savior of all mankind receives! Imagine sitting in a great concert hall and a world-class chorus is singing to the accompaniment of the finest orchestra in the world and they sing, "Blessing and honor, glory and power be unto Hutch [or your name]!" And just to make sure you heard them, they repeat that line over and over and over, concluding with one final phrase: For ever and ever!

For ever and ever!

As I sometimes have to say to my congregation, "You just missed an opportunity to say 'Amen!'" How short-sighted we are to hope for a pain-free life during our brief seventy- or eighty-year assignment on this planet. We measure our lives in days and months; God has plans for us that last for ever and ever. But there's more.

Why would he do that?

I don't know about you, but if all I got for my suffering was an eternity of receiving the same praise and admiration that Jesus receives from his Father, I don't think I'd ask another question.

"You mean I get to share in *your* glory, Jesus? You're God's Son. You sit right next to him and rule forever. I get a share of that? Awesome, God! Makes that throwing up I did throughout the night worth it."

If you look at your life from God's eternal perspective, you will feel exactly the same way about any misfortune you face. But sharing in his glory is a benefit or by-product of our suffering. It still doesn't explain *why* we have to go through these things.

In Romans 8:28–29, Paul has one more thing to say about our suffering, and it has to do with God's purpose for allowing us to go through difficult circumstances. It's the difference between *enduring* what we go through and *enjoying* it:

> And we know that in all things God works for the good of those who love him, who have been called according to his purpose. For those God foreknew he also predestined to be conformed to the likeness of his Son, that he might be the firstborn among many brothers. And those he predestined, he also called; those he called, he also justified; those he justified, he also glorified.
>
> Romans 8:28–30

God allows you to suffer because he wants you to be like Jesus. He will do whatever it takes to make you and me like Jesus, regardless of how much we cry, scream, get angry, or throw a fit. He is more interested in our character than our comfort, and he knows that becoming more like Jesus makes us more available for him to show other people what Christ is really like. God is more interested in his plan for all mankind than our plans for a good day. He is more interested in our holiness than our happiness, and if he's got to make us unhappy to make us holy, well, we better get ready to get rid of that smile for a while.

OK, maybe I got a little carried away with that last

statement, because God likes to see us smile, which is why we need to go back to two words from Romans 8:28: *all things*. When God inspired Paul and others who contributed to the Bible, he chose his words very carefully. Unlike me, he didn't need an editor to help him come up with the right words to make sure he wasn't being misunderstood. He could have said, "In *most* things God works for the good," but he said *all* things. Or he could have said, "In all the *good* things that happen to you God works for the good," but he said *all* things. That means good things, bad things, and everything in between.

So what are your "all things"? A bad marriage? A rebellious teenager who's in jail? A chronic condition such as diabetes? Bad credit? A boss who can't stand you because you're a Christian? No health insurance? You weren't paying attention and ran a stop sign and now the driver in the other car is paralyzed from the neck down and you're facing jail time?

These are some seriously bad things, but according to the Bible, God works in them for the good. It doesn't matter if the things that happen to you are fair or unfair. Your fault or someone else's. It doesn't matter if you were the driver or the victim; you're both experiencing something pretty awful — and if you've both been adopted into God's family, you can both say, "This is good."

Or you can complain. Shake your fist at God. Try to bargain with him. It doesn't matter to God, because the deal is already done. He has "predestined" you to become like Jesus, and he'll do whatever it takes, regardless of whether you like it or not. In a way, it's like when your six-year-old has a cold and the doctor prescribes medication to speed up his recovery. Your youngster doesn't want to take the medicine because it tastes bad. But it doesn't matter — you make him take that bitter medicine every day until the prescription runs out. You'd like him to be happier about it, but even if he's not, you still make him take it because you're more interested in him getting better than being happy.

Like a good father who wants the best for his child, God wants the best for us, and if that means allowing us to take the "medicine" that molds us into the likeness of his Son, why would he withhold that from us?

Of course, God would prefer that you trust his purpose and can therefore see the good in whatever you're going through. It is that trust that led James, who is thought to be the earthly brother of Jesus, to say it is "pure joy" to face "trials of many kinds" (James 1:2). Paul echoes this thought in his letter to the Romans: "We also rejoice in our sufferings, because we know that suffering produces perseverance; perseverance, character; and character, hope" (Romans 5:3–4).

I know this is tough teaching. It's counterintuitive to think of rejoicing when we suffer. But if we look at our lives from the perspective of the sovereign God, we see that ultimately our sufferings are what give us the kind of hope that keeps us going and that attracts others to us and to the faith we have embraced. When we think of the true heroes of the faith, they are people who have suffered greatly yet who see that their "all things" are good. The New Testament book of Hebrews list a virtual "hall of faith" of men and women who suffered greatly but knew their sufferings were all part of God's ultimate purpose — people "chained and put in prison ... stoned ... sawed in two ... put to death by the sword" (Hebrews 11:36 – 37). I'm reminded of a little book (now out of print) called *Prayers of the Martyrs* — and as the title suggests, the book contains the final prayers of men and women who have been killed for their belief in Christ.

One prayer in particular illustrates what happens when we understand God's purpose in allowing us to suffer: "Blessed are you, Lord Jesus Christ, Son of God, for you have, in your mercy, been so kind as to allow me a death like yours" (Papylus of Thyateira, died about AD 250).*

When we consider our unpleasant circumstances from a temporary, human perspective, God seems cruel or, at the very least, unconcerned about our suffering. But when we understand his purpose, we can begin to comprehend just how much he loves us — enough to follow through on his commitment to shape us into the character and likeness of Jesus. I'll never forget the letter I received from a woman, which illustrates so tenderly how there are no bad circum-

---

*Quoted in Duane W. H. Arnold, *Prayers of the Martyrs* (Grand Rapids: Zondervan, 1991), 78.

stances in the life of a Christian. She shared that her husband was being tested for Alzheimer's disease because he had been showing signs of memory loss and confusion. Of course, the idea of seeing her beloved husband sink deeper into dementia was devastating, but this dear woman understood that even this horrible news was made good by God: "While I pray for healing for my husband, I am also praying that I might surrender completely to God's will. Because of Jesus, I will be able to care for my husband, which will mold me more into a reflection of Christ."

I hate the idea of a little boy losing all his hair from chemotherapy and being so sick he can't play soccer. I hate the fact that I've had to miss some of my son's football games because I've been so weak I couldn't even sit up. Can you imagine what it must be like for a dad who used to be a professional football player not being able to watch his son play football? I'm human. When I'm hurting I cry like everyone else does. But through the tears, I can see another Father watching his Son carry his own cross to Calvary — and that's when I understand how something that seems so bad can be so good. I realize that it took my Lord's suffering to give me hope, and I see with fresh eyes that my own suffering is making me more and more like him.

I remember one dark night when I was in such intense pain that I didn't think I could take it anymore. Even with the powerful medication my doctor gave me to dull the pain, it wouldn't let up. Just kept getting worse and worse. I'd change positions to try to get more comfortable, but all that did was send me into convulsions. I've never really thought about giving up, but on that night I was ready for God to take me home so I could be rid of the pain once and for all. But just when I thought I couldn't handle it anymore, I started sobbing, not with the kind of tears that come from pain or despair, but with the kind of tears that automatically well up when someone out of the blue does something nice for you that you didn't expect and are quite sure you don't deserve. I was crying because I was so overwhelmed at the thought that God loved me with such a strong love that he would allow me to go through this night so that I could become more like his Son.

God is doing the same thing for you. Every inconvenience, every accident, every tragedy has a divine purpose. *All things.* To make you more and more like Jesus. To let you share in his glory. And, through it all, to attract more people to him.

What could be better than that?

It Only Looks Hopeless

If you are having trouble believing "it's all good," I don't blame you. For many of you—more than 15 million people as I write this—it's hard to believe because you're out of work. A great nation such as ours—with PhDs waiting in unemployment lines and applying for food stamps! Forget about the loss of income. Do you realize what it does to a man's or woman's self-esteem to be unemployed? Do you know how difficult and embarrassing it is for someone to stand in a long line at the unemployment office or to visit a food pantry?

I was told recently about a man who held the number two position in a medium-sized business related to the auto industry. Suddenly he found himself "downsized," that polite-sounding word that meant he wouldn't be getting a paycheck anymore. He sent his resume to more than fifty companies. He went to dozens of interviews, some in other

103

states, making the trip at his own expense and wondering how he was going to pay the credit card bill when it arrived at the end of the month. When his unemployment ran out, he had to accept financial assistance from his friends just to put food on the table. After eleven months without a job, he finally landed something: driving a school bus part-time at $11.70 an hour, with no health insurance or other benefits. He and his wife have two teenagers and a house on which they pay a sizable mortgage. You know what he said about the whole ordeal?

"The lack of money isn't the worst thing about losing your job. It's the feeling that you're worthless. You don't matter. No one wants you."

Now there's someone who could use some hope.

You might be one of the lucky ones who still has a job, but just how lucky are you? In this once prosperous and proud nation, workers are seeing their salaries capped or reduced as the cost of living skyrockets. Or they're losing benefits, such as health care, so they either have to pay for health insurance and other benefits out of their shrinking paychecks, or they drop their coverage and hope no one gets sick. Because so many of their colleagues got laid off, they have to work twice as hard to keep the business going. And because of all this, they're buying fewer cars, appliances, and clothes, which leads to more job losses at those and other businesses, despite billions of your dollars being spent to bail out the big spenders. Even as our nation's bankers saw the coming financial meltdown, they took greater risks by convincing millions of people they could afford huge houses beyond their means, thanks to "creative financing" that fueled outrageous salaries and gigantic bonuses being paid about the time those home-owners lost their homes.

Something tells me you're not too happy about the economy and could use some hope.

Have you checked your 401(k) lately? Like you, I joke about it. "Based on my retirement fund, I'm gonna have to work until I'm 103." But it's not a very funny joke. Baby boomers have lost billions of dollars they were counting on to help them live comfortably into their senior years. Look at the number of senior citizens working at McDonald's. You think they're taking your order because they've always longed for a career in fast food? They're trying to pay for the medicine they need to stay alive because Medicare is such a mess. I read recently that a lot of our senior citizens have to decide which of their prescriptions to buy because they can't afford all of them. Can you imagine having to choose between insulin and your blood pressure medicine? "Do I want a seizure or a stroke?"

This, by the way, isn't an indictment against any president or political party — Democrat, Republican, Independent. I'm not pointing fingers at any senator or governor — liberal, moderate, or conservative. For the most part, these are decent people trying hard to improve our lives, but it's not working. And if the economy is a mess, other corners of our culture are even more distressing.

For example, you don't have to be a preacher to be concerned about the moral condition in our nation. Think about it. By just about every poll or survey, between 75 and 85 percent of Americans see themselves as Christians. Of the remaining percentages, the majority adhere to other religions that teach strong family values, honesty, common decency, and sexual purity. Only about 4 percent of Americans describe themselves as atheists—but even atheists claim to have high moral standards.

Are you happy about the way our culture is living up to these moral standards?

I'm not. For example, we have one of the highest divorce rates in the world. And the difference in the divorce rate among regular churchgoers and the rest of the population is statistically negligible. Wouldn't you think a civilized nation where most of its citizens attend church or synagogue would have a little better record on marriage?

Speaking of marriage, if you're over forty, did you ever think that in your lifetime you would see pictures in the newspaper and on television of a man getting married to another man or a woman getting married to another woman? And did you think someone who raised a voice of protest against this would be publicly vilified and even physically threatened? Out where I live in the Pacific Northwest, there's a $1 million bounty on my head because of my public opposition to "gay marriage." To be fair, the bounty is not for someone to kill me, though I've faced enough threats of physical harm that I have to be careful. No, this bounty has been offered to anyone who can dig up some dirt to show everyone what a hypocrite I am. They figure if they can catch me in a compromising position, it will silence my criticism of gay marriage.

Is it any wonder so many good, decent people are losing hope? Who would have thought you could get in trouble for standing up for what's right?

Here's another one I just can't figure out. How can a society in which the vast majority of people believe that Jesus is the Son of God allow more than one million abortions each year? In 2006, Planned Parenthood, which identifies itself as "the nation's leading sexual and reproductive health care provider," performed 289,750 abortions at its clinics, a new record for them. That is, until they released their numbers for 2007: 305,310, an increase of 5 percent. I'm sure you're as disheartened as I am about the work of Planned Parenthood, especially when you realize we're helping to pay for it: 34 percent of Planned Parenthood's overall budget comes from our taxes!

What do you think would happen if a construction project would kill even just a few dozen lives of a protected species such as the ivory-billed woodpecker or the California tiger salamander? You'd have hundreds of protesters picketing the job site, and maybe even people engaging in some criminal activity by trying to stop the bulldozers from destroying the habitat for one of these endangered species. Now I love animals. I live in a rural area east of Seattle and marvel at the birds and deer and delicate plants that make up our ecosystem. But are they more valuable than a little baby inside a mama's belly? And yet, when God-honoring people like you and me speak out against abortion, we're labeled as irrational radicals — religious fundamentalists along the lines of the Taliban.

Where's the hope for a little baby who has been innocently enjoying her home inside her mother's womb for three months?

Isn't it amazing how things that once were considered offensive are now part of the mainstream? When I was a rebellious teenager growing up in the 1960s, you had to really work at getting your hands on a copy of a magazine like *Playboy*. Pornography in America has become a nearly $15 billion business, making it a bigger business than professional football, basketball, and baseball combined.* The 4.2 million pornographic websites on the Internet generate 68 million search engine requests every day, and a shocking 116,000 of those requests are for *child* pornography.** By the

---

*Cited in Frank Rich, "Naked Capitalists: There's No Business Like Porn Business," *New York Times* magazine (May 20, 2001), *http://www.nytimes.com/2001/05/20/magazine/20PORN.html?pagewanted=all*.

**Cited in Jerry Ropelato, "Internet Pornography Statistics," Internet Filter Review, Top Ten Reviews, *http://internet-filter-review.toptenreviews.com/internet-pornography-statistics.html*.

way, I don't know of any God-fearing person who thinks pornography is a good thing, so who's typing in "porn" on their search engines 68 million times a day?

"Hey Hutch? I thought this was a book about hope. You've quit preaching and started meddling!"

You must have been talking to the people at my church. They probably warned you, "That guy's crazy! He actually believes every word in the Bible." Sometimes I feel sorry for those dear people at my church because they got *me* for a pastor. They could easily find churches where preachers pick and choose which parts of the Bible are worth paying attention to. I believe everything the Bible teaches, but our people still come every Sunday. Let me tell you, they've got to really *want* to come to my church because there's nothing convenient about it. My priorities as a minister have always been people first, then programs, and finally facilities. So all of our money goes into helping people and implementing programs that change and improve their lives — and whatever is left over goes to renting whatever building we can find. It takes seven trailers and a lot of volunteers just to set up our rental building for church each Sunday. And sometimes we've been kicked out of buildings because of my views, which I can't claim to have thought up on my own since they come straight from the Bible.

And to make matters worse, I really don't care if the people at my church like me or not. I mean, I'm human. Of course I want to be liked. Who doesn't? But if being liked means lying to them, I just can't do it. I have to tell them the truth because I honestly believe that's what gives them hope for a better life. That truth is what allows me to live with the pain and discomfort of cancer and consider it a good thing instead of a burden to bear.

It's that same truth that will give you the hope you need to live the life you've always wanted to live.

Can't We All Just Be Tolerant?

We live in a world where a lot of good, decent people appear to have given up. That's the only way I can explain some of these things that are going on in our world. I'm sure you don't like what's happening in our culture any more than I do, but you've resigned yourself to thinking this is just the way it's going to be. That this is as good as it gets. Or you've been conditioned by the view that you're supposed to mind your own business. In our culture of so many different thoughts and beliefs, people are going to do things you disagree with, but you have no right to tell them it's wrong. And so you go along with that view on the surface, but deep inside you feel resentful. Maybe even a little angry.

You don't like having to worry about your kids turning on the television during "family viewing hours" and seeing programs that make adultery seem funny and normal. You think it's shameful that the teacher in your daughter's sex education class teaches her that homosexuality is normal or that it's OK for her to have sex with a guy as long as she insists he use a condom. You're tired of seeing more and more of the taxes you pay go to things you believe are wrong. But at the end of the day, you just tolerate it because, well, we're *supposed* to be tolerant. Besides, you don't see any evidence that anything will change, so why bother?

If this describes how you're feeling, then you need a good dose of hope. Throughout this book, I've tried to show you where to find such hope and how to claim it as your own. You have seen that real hope can only be based on truth. You can't put your hope in a lie. And the truth is that no government or political party or law is going to change the things that are causing you to lose hope for a better life. The answer to our problems won't be found in Washington, D.C. That's not a criticism of any politician — just the truth. I don't blame any president, past or present, for promising that things will get better. I'm sure they meant well, but there's no way they can deliver, just as there's no way my doctor can give me a 100 percent guarantee that this cancer of mine will be cured. When he prescribes a new treatment, I know he wants it to work, but he can't promise me it will. He might say something like, "Thirty percent of the patients who have tried this new therapy have been in remission for an average of five years." Not bad. Thirty percent. Five years. I'll take it.

But wouldn't you rather put your hope in something that is guaranteed to work 100 percent of the time? Hope that doesn't depend on a bill passing in Congress or a big jump in the stock market? That's the kind of hope God offers us. In the face of all these things (and more) that drag us down, you can have the life you always wanted. A life that triumphs over *any* circumstance. A life that lets you look into the jaws of any illness, financial calamity, or family tragedy and say, "It's good."

If that's the kind of hope you really want, then I have a question for you: Whom are you going to trust?

You Can't Always Get What You Want

In the real-life story of Tyler Doughtie — the story that inspired the making of the movie *Letters to God*, Tyler's family and friends prayed that God would heal him. But God chose not to. From the day I was diagnosed with my own cancer, I have been asking God to heal me. I've still got cancer, and it's worse now than it was when I started praying.

Sometimes it's not the circumstances of your life that get you down; it's the sneaking suspicion that God doesn't care about you. It feels like he's ignoring you. You pray your little heart out for him to do something, and you get nothing. I'm not even talking only about big miracles or anything like that, but those prayers where you ask him to help you find a job or make your marriage work better. And after weeks or even months of that same prayer, you still don't have a job, or you and your wife are still barely tolerating each other.

So here's the question: How can you have hope when God doesn't even seem to be listening to you?

I heard about a guy whose fifteen-year-old daughter ran away from home, and, of course, it just devastated him. This guy was a fired-up Christian so he did what every Christian is taught to do when tragedy strikes: he prayed that God would send his daughter back to him. I don't mean he just said a little prayer and went about his business. He *really* prayed. Every morning when he woke up, it was the first thing he did, sometimes actually lying flat on his face in his bedroom, crying out to God. He prayed on the way to work and on the drive back home, and he ended every day praying until he fell asleep. If anyone ever followed the biblical instruction to "pray without ceasing," this guy came pretty close. The last I heard, he had kept praying like that for more than a year — and still no sign of his daughter. You know what he said when a friend told him he should start to accept the fact that she was never coming back?

"Oh, I already have, but I don't know if God has, and until I know for a fact that she won't come back, I'm going to keep praying."

I don't know this man, but he's my kind of guy! Or more accurately, he's God's kind of guy. He understands an important truth that allows him to have hope, no matter what. He knows that God never makes a mistake and that whatever God chooses to do regarding his daughter is what's best. We so often make the mistake of thinking that if we don't get what we ask for, God must not care about us. Nothing in the Bible supports that. To the contrary, God loves us so much that he gives us what we need, even if it's not what we want. And he does it at exactly the perfect time.

Would Jesus Dis a Woman?

If anyone had a right to think that God had abandoned her, it was a woman in the New Testament known only as "a Canaanite woman." She doesn't even get a name in the Bible, and her story consumes all of seven brief verses. It's so short that unless you're specifically looking for it, you might miss it. But it's a powerful example of perseverance in the face of what can only be called rejection by God. At least that's what it felt like.

We learn about this woman in the gospel of Matthew, and her encounter with Jesus occurred at a time when Jesus was worn-out, physically and emotionally. Even though Jesus was the Son of God, he was fully human during his thirty-three years on earth, and we see that human side in this story. To set the stage, Jesus had received some really bad news. His friend John, who had baptized him, had been beheaded (Matthew 14:10). It was particularly distressing because Herod's wife had tricked her husband, who was the ruler of the region, into having him killed. Understandably,

Jesus wanted to be alone to absorb this horrible news. He's human, so he's sad and grieving and wants some time to himself.

But the word spread that Jesus was in the area, and literally thousands of people tracked him down because they had heard of his remarkable healing powers. Despite his sadness, he spent most of the day ministering to the people until his disciples suggested he send the crowd packing because night was approaching, the people were hungry, and there was no food in sight. But Jesus refused to turn the crowd away and instead fed the entire multitude with only five loaves of bread and two fish (Matthew 14:17).

Then he had a run-in with the religious leaders who had been stalking him, just waiting to catch him in some wrongdoing. You see, Jesus was a threat to the religious establishment. Just about everything he taught went against their own teaching, and what's worse, the people were being drawn to Jesus' message instead of theirs. So wherever he went he could count on a few spies being planted in the crowd to report back to the authorities. This time, they accused his disciples of not washing their hands before they ate. They had violated one of the hundreds of laws that Jewish people believed were necessary to obey in order to please God.

It is clear from Jesus' response to their accusation that he was quite annoyed at this petty charge. In fact, it's from this exchange between him and the religious leaders

(Matthew 15:14) that we get the phrase "the blind leading the blind." That shut them up, but Jesus still needed to find some downtime, so he headed to another mountain in an area inhabited primarily by Gentiles, probably thinking that none of the Jewish leaders would follow him into territory they considered unclean. And that's where he is confronted by the woman who is only identified by the region she came from—Canaan.

She was desperate, and here's how I know that. As a resident of Canaan, she would have been a Gentile. Jesus was a Jew. The relationship between Jews and Gentiles at the time was such that they kept their distance from each other. It's not overstating things to say they hated each other. As far as this woman knew, Jesus was a Jewish man who helped people, and she needed help. So she swallowed her pride and approached Jesus. Totally humbled herself and made herself vulnerable in the presence of this group of Jewish men. It would be a little bit like a black slave woman in the 1850s walking right up to the richest white man in town and asking for help—only worse. So this woman must have been at the end of her rope to approach a Jewish man, and we learn that yes, indeed, she was: "Lord, Son of David, have mercy on me! My daughter is suffering terribly from demon-possession" (Matthew 15:22).

In that brief request, she addresses him as a superior (Lord), acknowledges that he is the Jewish Messiah (Son of David), and then begs for help. If any other Gentiles in the area were to hear her call a Jew by the title of Lord, they would have disowned her and quite likely punished her. That's desperation, but if you're a mom and you've ever had a little daughter who needed help, you understand.

So there it is. Her plea echoes in the air.

And Jesus ignored her.

Jesus, the Son of a loving God, the miracle man well-known in the area for healing children and reaching out to the poor and oppressed. Refused to even notice her. In my neighborhood, we call that "dissing" someone. Big-time.

Have you ever been dissed? Have you ever made yourself vulnerable to someone and had them totally ignore and reject you? I know a man who struggled with an addiction to pornography. He attended a big church. He was in a small group, and one day he decided to share his struggle with his group of caring Christians. He told a bit of his story, and there was silence. Silence. He says he felt like he had leprosy. No one said a word to him after that. Guys who used to invite him to play golf—well, they quit calling. So he stopped going to that church—and I don't blame him, just as I wouldn't blame the Canaanite woman if she had turned her back on Jesus. But she didn't.

This Gentile woman who was just dissed by the Son of God persisted, even after Jesus told her that his mission really was only for the Jews—that giving the Bread of Life to a Gentile would be the same as tossing it to the dogs. In so many words he was saying to this desperate woman,

"Look, I'm here to take care of the Jews. Nothing personal, but if I help you, it would be like tossing a loaf of bread to the dogs." That's right. Jesus called this woman a dog! This is absolutely true; it's right there in the Bible. What was he thinking?

Undeterred, this desperate mother knelt down before Jesus and told him she understood she didn't deserve his help but was willing to settle for crumbs. Only then did Jesus answer her: "Woman, you have great faith! Your request is granted" (Matthew 15:28). And the Bible says that her daughter was healed at that very moment.

Drive-up Christianity

I'm guessing you may never have heard this story of the Canaanite woman. If you have, you probably haven't heard many sermons on it. And if you have heard a sermon on it, you were probably told that Jesus wanted to see what the woman was going to do — that he wanted to see if she would persevere. Whoever told you that has a pretty lousy view of God. And an incorrect one at that! That interpretation implies that God really doesn't know what he's doing — that he's making it up as he goes along. Even worse, this picture of God paints him as some sort of mad scientist, testing the limits of this poor woman to see how much she can take. Would *you* trust a God like that?

The Bible teaches that God knows everything. He knew exactly what that woman would do. He wanted *her* to

know what she was going to do. To find out for herself what
she was made of. He wanted her to discover she could go
a lot further than she thought. It wasn't a test of her faith
but a revelation. From the human perspective, Jesus walked
right by that woman, ignoring her and not caring about her
one iota. From an eternal perspective—one that declares
God as sovereign—he was saying, "Come on, honey. Follow
me. Keep asking. You're not going to believe how strong you
are. Your daughter is going to be fine. And so are you."

I used to hate doing wind sprints at the end of football
practice. We had just gone at it hard and heavy for two
hours, and then the coach blew his whistle and made us
line up on the goal line. The next whistle meant we had
to sprint the length of the field, turn around, line up on
that goal line, and in about five seconds take off running
to the next whistle. You know how hot it gets in Alabama
in August? Hot enough to turn the humid air into steam.
But he just kept blowing the whistle and we kept running
until we thought we couldn't go on, and then he'd make us
run one more sprint. Always one more than we thought
we could do. *He* knew we could do it, but we didn't. He
was showing us what we were made of, and that's exactly
what Jesus was doing for the Canaanite woman. He saw the
future and knew there would be a time when she would face
something even bigger than the death of her daughter, and
he wanted her to know she could face *anything*.

What would have happened if this woman who took

such a risk in approaching Jesus had given up after he
ignored her? The obvious result is she would still have a
child who was sick and demon-possessed. But she also would
have left the scene with a defeated spirit. "What a fool I am!
I never should have trusted a Jew to pay attention to me."
And she never would have learned how strong she was. An
experience like this would have set the trajectory for the
rest of her life. We never hear a word about her after this
story, but what do you think it did for her to hang in there,
in spite of what appeared to be a thorough dissing from
Jesus? I'm guessing she not only went away and told all of
her Gentile friends about Jesus but also faced the rest of her
life with enormous confidence and trust in God.

When I first decided to fight my cancer, I couldn't
understand why God wouldn't just heal me. I *believed* he
could and *asked* him to, but nothing happened — except
I just got sicker and weaker. I know a little bit about how
it feels to not hear from God. You feel lonely. Forgotten.
Unimportant. You feel as if God has much bigger things to
do than to help you, and you even feel like giving up. Now
as I think back on those experiences, I'm so glad God let
me go through the valley because he taught me so much
through it all. You've probably heard people who've gone
through rough times say they were the best times of their
lives. It's true. While I would never wish the pain and sense
of abandonment I felt on anyone, I have to say those were
some of the best days of my life. As a result, what I believed

in my head became implanted on my heart: *All* things are good if you love Jesus.

When it seems as though God is ignoring us, most of us just give up too soon. We treat Christianity like a drive-up window, and we don't even want to slow down to pick up our food! But Jesus is saying to us, "You have to stick around long enough to see what I'm cooking. Don't settle for a hamburger when I'm working on a gourmet meal. Shut your engine off. Come on inside and sit down. Sometimes good food takes time."

You will have many times in your life when it seems as if God has just walked right on past you when you called on him for help. You've been praying for something important, and he just doesn't seem to be paying attention. Few things feel worse than being abandoned by a friend or a loved one, but God *never* abandons his children. *Never*. When you can't understand the hand of God, trust his face. When you can't understand why he seems so silent, trust his character. God is love, but sometimes it's tough love so that you get the best instead of the better. He knows what you need to have the life that brings you the greatest good, and most of the time it's not what you're asking for. In fact, he knows that if you always got what you asked for, your life would be a mess.

When I was playing in the NFL, I saw what happened when guys who grew up having nothing could have everything they ever wanted. They would sign these huge contracts right out of college that gave them more money than they had ever seen in their lives. And within a few years, these guys were gone. Out of football, out of money, and out of luck. They thought they knew what they needed. Fancy cars. Big houses. Bling. Women whenever they wanted one. What most of us would consider "the good life." If I hadn't already settled the question of who was sovereign, I might have done the same thing.

Sometimes it's good not to get what you want, especially if what you want is not what God wants for you. You might think you want a better-paying job, but God can see into the future, and he knows that the job you want will give you more stress than you can handle, keep you away from your family when they need you, or maybe even put you first in line when your company has to cut back. It will give you more money, but you'll take the stress home with you and it will mess with your family. It might be a good job. It might be better than your current job. But it's not the *best* for you, and God wants you to have the best! He's willing to let you deal with a little disappointment in order to give you the best.

So no matter how hard you pray for that new job and it just doesn't happen, don't get discouraged. Trust God and be thankful that not only is he giving you the best; he is molding you to be like Jesus in the process. Some people might look at me and think I missed out by not enjoying all the "fun" that was available to me as a football player, but who do you think is having more fun—that guy sitting by himself in an apartment trying to figure out where his life went, or me?

Never Let Go of the End of a Rope

There's one more lesson from this story of the woman with no name—the Gentile woman who dared to approach the Jewish Messiah and got insulted for her efforts, the woman Jesus called a dog. She came to Jesus because she was desperate. She had no other place to go, no one else to turn to. She was on a mission to save her daughter, and she would not be deterred. She had obviously heard about Jesus and had complete trust that he could help her. When he ignored her, she didn't know why. She had no clue what was going on, but she didn't need to. When he told her he was there to help the Jews instead of the Gentiles, she might have been puzzled, but she didn't argue with him. And when he called her a dog, it must have hurt, but she didn't protest. She went with the program because, despite all she didn't know or couldn't understand, she knew one thing: this was Jesus. I can almost hear her saying to herself, "I don't have to understand him. I don't have to figure out what he's doing. But I know who he is, and that's enough. I know I can trust Jesus."

Most of us let go when we get to the end of our rope. We've reasoned with God. Bargained with him. Made promises to him. Begged him, and he still hasn't come through. So we conclude that God doesn't care, and we let go of the rope. This woman refused to let go, and it saved her daughter. To our way of thinking, it doesn't make sense, but the greater the suffering that God allows you to experience, the greater the blessing when he does come through. And he always does.

Several years ago, a brilliant young man received his PhD and began teaching at a major university. Raised in a home that honored God, he turned his back on his parents' faith, ultimately declaring that he was an atheist. As he climbed the academic ladder he began drinking heavily. His marriage began to suffer, and he was on a path to personal and spiritual ruin.

A family friend began praying for this man when he began his teaching career. She saw the direction his life was going and how he had completely rejected God, so she started praying. Every day she prayed the same prayer — that this man would turn his life over to Jesus. The more she prayed, the deeper he sank into a pattern of abusive behavior toward his family and himself. Yet she kept praying — twenty-two years of praying the same prayer every day. And then finally the man humbled himself before God, confessed his sins, and accepted the gift of salvation.

When you get a chance, type the name "Lyle W. Dorsett" into your computer's search engine. You'll see that he's an evangelist, a prolific author of books on prayer and evangelism, and the Billy Graham professor of evangelism at a prominent Christian seminary. I'm sure that one lone persistent woman who prayed for him for so long couldn't have understood why God kept ignoring her. I'm guessing there were days when she felt it was useless, a complete waste of time, to keep on praying—that maybe God had other plans and that she should turn her focus to something else. But she just kept on praying for Lyle Dorsett.

What do you think would have happened if she had given up after a couple of years? God in his providence might have still captured the heart of Lyle Dorsett. That would have been good. That woman might have begun praying for someone else, and that would have been good too. The truth is, God always gives us his best. For reasons we may not understand, God chose to let this woman pray for twenty-two years, but it produced an evangelist who has preached to thousands and has influenced hundreds of students to devote themselves to ministry. All because a woman trusted God when it looked as though God was passing her by.

Are You Feeling Dissed?

I believe God can do anything. The Bible teaches that he is all-powerful, which means there is nothing he is not capable of doing. It is because I believe this that I pray confidently every day that God will heal me of this annoying disease. So far he hasn't. When my doctor recommends a new treatment that might wipe out my cancer, I go for it, even though I know the side effects will lay me low for a while. As the new treatment starts, I pray that God will use it to defeat the cancer. And I confidently await the results after the treatment is finished. Maybe this time he will use the science and technology he has given the medical field. But after each new regimen, the cancer is still there.

Does that mean he has forgotten about me or that he just doesn't care whether I get better or not? Not at all. I want to get better, but he wants the best. If I have to suffer a little in order to get the best, sign me up, because God's best is beyond anything I could possibly imagine.

Is there something you've been asking God to do and he hasn't done it yet? Are you tempted to give up hope because God hasn't answered your prayers? Then you're in the perfect place for a great blessing. Maybe not tomorrow. Or the next day. But God *will* come through, regardless of how you feel, because he's all you got. He's all you need.

He's the only one who can give you the best.

No Fear

If I asked you to tell me in one word what the opposite of *hope* is, you would probably say *hopelessness*. And you'd be right. But that's too easy. So describe the opposite of hope in one word without using any form of the word *hope*. Despair? Disillusionment? Resignation? Those are all great answers that describe exactly what happens when you do not have hope. But when I see someone who has lost hope, what I really see is someone who has let *fear* take over. And as I observe the way so many decent people in our society are living, I see a lot of fearful people.

Here's just a partial list of the things we're afraid of:

I'm afraid I'm going to lose my job.

I already lost my job; now I'm afraid I'm going to lose my house.

I'm afraid my kids are going to use drugs.

I'm afraid of the kinds of people who are moving into my neighborhood.

I'm afraid my taxes are going to go up.

I'm afraid I won't be able to afford to send my kids
 to college.
I'm afraid of a terrorist attack.
I'm afraid to get married because most marriages
 don't work.
I'm afraid someone is going to steal my identity.
I'm afraid of getting swine flu.
I'm afraid my beliefs will offend my friends.
I'm afraid of global warming.
I'm afraid my spouse might leave me.
I'm afraid I won't have enough money to retire.
I'm afraid of what my kids are learning in public schools.
I'm afraid we might run out of oil.
I'm afraid I'll get cancer.

Fear is such a debilitating force in our lives. It just sort
of sits on our shoulders telling us that things are going to be
bad. It's like a thief, robbing us of the life we were intended
to live — a life filled with eager anticipation for whatever
is around the next turn. I'm reminded of a married couple
who has basically lived their lives in fear. When they got
married, they were afraid to have kids because they were
fearful of trying to raise kids in a world that they thought
was, well, fearful. When their kids were little they were constantly afraid they would get hurt, and so they spent most of
their time trying to protect their kids from the usual bumps
and bruises that go along with being a kid. (I mean, come

on, if you don't get at least one set of stitches when you're a kid, you aren't living.) When their kids were teenagers, they began to worry about who they would marry. After their two kids grew up and married wonderful spouses, they were afraid their marriages wouldn't last. Now they're in their fifties, and all they can talk about is how old they are, how they might not have enough money to retire, and what they're going to do if they can't take care of themselves. Chances are they're going to live for at least another twenty years — twenty more years of being scared — and then what?

What a horrible way to live, especially for a couple who goes to church every Sunday, reads the Bible, and prays every day. I can almost imagine their prayers: "Oh, God, please let me hang on for another day." And that's pretty much what they're doing. Hanging on.

Play as if the Game Has Been Won

The Bible has a lot to say about fear. (Actually it has only one thing to say about fear, but it repeats it a lot.) Find a copy of the New International Version of the Bible and start counting every verse that mentions fear or being afraid. It will be a lot easier if you get an electronic version and download it to your computer. That way you can just type the words *fear*, *fears*, *feared*, and *afraid* into the search function and the results will pop right up! Look at the Hutch — going all digital on you!

Here's what you will find:

"do not be afraid" (65 times)
"don't be afraid" (24 times)
"do not fear" (18 times)
"have no fear" (4 times)
"do not be fainthearted or afraid" (1 time)
"do not lose heart or be afraid" (1 time)
"do not give way to fear" (1 time)
"fear not" (1 time)

Anytime somebody repeats something 115 times, it's gotta be pretty important. You think God's trying to tell you something? Absolutely! God knows that you cannot enjoy the life he created for you if you're a big worrier. He knows how much you will miss out on the good things he has for you if you're afraid to venture out of your cocoon. Fear causes you to endure, while hope gives you the courage to live your life to the fullest. We are drawn to Tyler in *Letters to God* because he didn't let his disease diminish his enthusiasm for life. He knew what the score was in terms of life and death, but he chose to live life to the fullest. When he had a chance to play soccer with the team, he went for it, despite the risks to his weakened body.

As an athlete, I learned something about fear: If you play afraid, you'll get hurt. Even if you're fifty pounds heavier than the running back you have to tackle, if you head into that collision afraid it's going to hurt, it will. The best advice I ever got as a football player was to play as if you know you're going to win. There's nothing like the hope of victory to give you courage. So even if you go into the game as a three-touchdown underdog, play as though you will be walking off the field at the end of the game as the winning team. Approach a game with fear, and you're probably going to lose; run onto the field believing you will win, and at least you've got a fighting chance.

When quarterback Eli Manning took his New York Giants into the 2008 Super Bowl, few football fans gave them much of a chance to beat the 2006 Super Bowl champions, the New England Patriots. Every Friday before the Super Bowl, my good friend Rush Limbaugh calls me on the air, and we make our picks for the big game. Rush gave me a pretty hard time because I picked the Giants to win. We went at it pretty good, with Rush telling me all the reasons why the Patriots would easily win. At least a few journalists must have been listening to his show because the next day a sports writer said I was "stupid" for picking the Giants. On paper they were clearly the underdog, with many sports writers questioning Manning's leadership and skills. But in one of the most exciting Super Bowls in the game's history, the Giants were behind late in the game, and a Patriot victory seemed certain. With time running out and facing a ferocious blitz by the New England defense, Manning calmly found wide receiver Plaxico Burress all alone behind the defense and hit him with a pass that won the game.

"We never had doubt," he told reporters after the game. "We had total faith in ourselves, and we believed we could win, and we earned it."

When asked if he had any doubts they could come back to win after New England got off to a quick 14–0 lead, he answered, "No, we believed in ourselves all year."

Here's what I find so amazing about this story—in fact, about every story that tells of amazing comebacks by underdogs. Every rational piece of information tells them they cannot win. The other team is bigger, faster, stronger. They have more talented athletes. They have the momentum that comes from having a winning season. The cards are completely stacked against them, yet they enter the game believing they will win. Not that they *could* win or *might* win, but that they *will* win.

Which makes me wonder: Why do so many church folk live such fearful lives? We know the outcome. We're already on the winning side. We don't have to convince ourselves we're going to win; we *know* we will win. According to the Bible, God has set in motion a plan that will culminate in a complete victory over evil, culminating in the establishment of his eternal kingdom. When you committed your life to Jesus, you joined the winning team. Nothing can defeat you. The Bible doesn't mince words about this. It doesn't say we will win *most* of the time. Just as Saint Paul reminds us that *all* things turn out to be good for followers of Jesus, he tells us that we will be victorious in "all these things" (Romans 8:37).

In this passage in Romans, Paul asks a rhetorical question that sounds a lot like a locker-room pep talk: "If God is for us, who can be against us?" (Romans 8:31). Think about that for a moment. I can almost imagine the New York Giants' coach in the locker room before the Super Bowl: "Hey, we've got Eli Manning on our side. How can we possibly lose?" Except that Eli Manning is human. We have the Creator of the universe on our side, and not only that, but he's *for* us. Everything he does, every part of his eternal plan, has the goal of delivering to us a great and victorious life. How can we lose?

Then this great apostle gets specific and begins to name the enemies we might be afraid of: trouble, hardship, persecution, famine, nakedness, danger, swords.

That pretty much covers anything you and I will ever encounter in our lifetimes. You get behind in your mortgage? You're still on the winning side. Can't feed your family? You still win. People make fun of you because you take a stand for what you believe? Guess what — you win. An invading army takes over and kills you for your beliefs? You win, and they lose!

But just to make sure there's no confusion about the life God gives us, Paul continues:

> No, in all these things we are more than conquerors through him who loved us. For I am convinced that neither death nor life, neither angels nor demons, neither the present nor the future, nor

any powers, neither height nor depth, nor anything
else in all creation, will be able to separate us from
the love of God that is in Christ Jesus our Lord.

Romans 8:37–39

That means Islamic terrorists won't win. Laws that
legalize immoral behavior won't win. Incurable diseases
won't win. Hurricanes and global warming won't win. There
isn't a single thing in all creation that will be able to defeat
us. By the end of the game, we win!

When you consider the fact that we know we're going
to win, along with the dozens of messages from God that
tell us not to be afraid, why do so many of us hunker down
along the sidelines, afraid to get into the game? Why do so
many of us live timid lives, wringing our hands and whining about how bad things are? We have such a great and
real hope that ought to make us the most confident and
happy people on earth, but we act as though the situation
is hopeless.

What's So Bad about Winning?

I know that some people don't like to think of life in
terms of competition — in terms of winning or losing. It
doesn't seem "spiritual" to view life that way. That's OK for
sports or politics or wars, but when it comes to how I live
my life, can't everybody win? Do we have to consider those
who don't believe the way we do as enemies?

These people fail to understand that you can't escape

the battle between good and evil. You're in it every day, whether you like it or not. The reason you feel so helpless so much of the time is that you're living by your wishes, not by your beliefs. The Bible makes it very clear that the forces of good and evil are constantly at war. You have the choice of joining the winning side and helping fight evil, sticking with the losers, or trying to remain neutral. Jesus had something to say about trying to be neutral. He pictured it as lukewarm water. Have you ever reached for a glass of water (you were expecting cold water), and after taking a gulp, you realized it was lukewarm? Or you grabbed your cup of coffee and instead of a steaming mug of your favorite blend, it was barely warm? Jesus was writing to a group of Christians who refused to take a stand for their faith and said, "Because you are lukewarm — neither hot nor cold — I am about to spit you out of my mouth" (Revelation 3:16).

You don't want God to spit you out, do you?

There is no in-between with God. You are either for him or against him. Trying to be neutral so that everybody likes you is the same as being against him. A lot of church folk get all religious and righteous when everything is going well, but when it comes time to do battle, they become lukewarm. You know why? They're afraid.

In 2004, I learned just how afraid some of these church folk are. If you haven't guessed by now, I'm sort of an activist. When I see something that needs fixing, I try to fix it, and one of the things that needs fixing is the way we think about marriage. As you know, some people want everyone to believe that marriage should be redefined to include people of the same gender, making it legal for men to marry men and women to marry women. I disagree and thought it would be a good idea to invite people in my home state of Washington to gather at our big stadium, Safeco Field, to show our governor and legislators that we don't want marriage defined in that way. So I started making phone calls and invited as many church leaders as I could find to join me in planning what I was calling Mayday for Marriage.

First I was told I would never get an open date at Safeco Field. I checked, and they had just one opening — in just thirty days. Then I was told there was no way we could organize this type of event with only thirty days to prepare for it. When I pushed back, the real reasons started coming out: We'll look like fools. It will just antagonize people. We won't be able to pay for it. No one will show up. No one came right out and said it, but they were afraid. Thankfully, enough leaders knew they were on the winning team and simply believed it would happen. They knew that with a sovereign God, anything is possible. In fact, if you break apart the word *impossible* and add an apostrophe, you get a description of God: *I'm possible.*

More than 20,000 people showed up and we had a great time celebrating God's design for marriage.

So I decided to try the same thing on a national level and started planning an event in Washington, D.C. Once again, I discovered how foolish and naive I was, as national church leaders, many of whose names you would recognize, called and tried to talk me out of it. Only five people eventually joined me in planning this national Mayday for Marriage event, and two months before it was scheduled to take place, we started getting calls from prominent Christian leaders asking us to call it off. They said it would be impossible to draw a significant crowd to Washington, D.C., and that we would embarrass the church if we went ahead with it. As an African American, I know what it means to stand up for something you believe in — something that's right in God's eyes, no matter who says it isn't. God has put us here as the salt of the earth. No other institution, no other people group, is called the bride of Christ except the church. If we don't stand up for what God has ordained, who will?

More than 250,000 people from all over the country descended on the Mall in our nation's capital to stand up for God's design for marriage, despite the fact that it was a rainy day. In fact, the more it rained, the more people came out. Impossible? Embarrassing? Hardly. As one news source reported, "The immense support for pro-marriage legislation was reflected by the crowds of people who traveled from near and far to stand among those who believe strongly, like themselves, in the sanctity of marriage."* I'm

---

*PR Newswire, "Tens of Thousands Flock to D.C. in Defense of Traditional Marriage" (October 15, 2004).

sure some of those who wanted to call this event off were worried about the media making the event look bad, but is that any reason to retreat from what you know is right? And as it turned out, *The Village Voice*, usually known for unflattering coverage of Christian ideas, gave it the fairest and most accurate treatment of anyone.

Of all the leaders I contacted to help us with this event, only five dared hope that God would come through, but that was enough. The rest let fear cloud their vision.

Numbers don't mean anything to God. One skinny kid with a slingshot killed Goliath with one pebble. Gideon routed thousands of heavily armed Midianites with only three hundred men armed with trumpets and torches. Daniel stood all by himself in a den of lions. Jesus began a worldwide movement with only twelve followers. If God wants to do something, he doesn't worry about the opposition.

How would your life be different if instead of being afraid to do something, you dared to put your hope in the God who has already won? I'm talking not just about big moral issues that are destroying our culture but everyday things you and I face. One of the ministries of our church that I'm extremely proud of is called Antioch Adoptions. It grew out of a burden to see all the foster children in our area become adopted into "forever homes." We wanted to remove as many barriers as possible to help families adopt these children, but we didn't have the money to fund the program. At first I was a little worried about how we would come up with the money, but I came back to my "spiritual senses" and realized that if God is behind something, I don't need to be afraid of doing it. So after preaching on the parable of the talents, we gave everyone over eighteen a ten dollar bill—doling out a total of $20,000. Six months later, they returned the ten dollars, along with whatever they earned from that investment, and we collected $280,000, enough to open our center with a full-time professional staff. We now place between thirty and forty children into adoptive families each year.

Now here's the cool part. Our adoption program has gotten quite a bit of attention, which has encouraged others to consider adopting as well. Here's just one of the emails I've received from courageous adoptive parents:

> I'm a white adoptive mom of two of the most beautiful black children you've ever seen! Not only that, but I deal with life from a wheelchair due to muscular dystrophy. My kids don't suffer because of it; in fact, God's grace covers them so uniquely that I wonder at his works. I have no fear of man, chemotherapy, or the future. My times are in his hands.

Wow! Imagine what might never have happened if I had let my fear about money direct my steps. Imagine how you might be missing out on God's absolute best because of your fears. Some parents are afraid to talk with their kids about drugs or sex, when they should relax and trust the fact that God's way will prevail if they give it a chance. Besides, if you aren't talking to your kids about these things, who is? Are you comfortable with them being taught by someone who doesn't honor God? Maybe you've always wanted to change jobs or go back to school or send your kids to another school, but you were afraid of what might happen. Let me assure you, if God is telling you to do something, you don't ever have to be afraid. If your motive for doing something is to honor God, you can't lose.

Onward, Christian Wimps

We used to sing an old hymn called "Onward, Christian Soldiers" that depicted Christians as "marching on to war." Given the disappointing wars we have fought in since Vietnam, the song seems to have lost its popularity. And in our well-intentioned efforts to not offend anyone, we don't like to be thought of as soldiers. We want to be liked, and we especially don't want any individual to think we hate them for what they believe or don't believe. But that old hymn got it right. We *are* in a war, not against other people — because God loves everyone — but against ideas and practices that violate God's ways and threaten to destroy the very people who embrace them. But it's a war that has already been won. So why fight so timidly? Why be so apologetic for fighting for the winning team?

Throughout the course of human history, there have been only four world kingdoms: Babylonian, Persian, Greek, and Roman. As each kingdom advanced on other regimes in order to conquer them, they first sent their ambassadors to announce the impending takeover. These kingdom ambassadors always entered the new territory with power, strength, and courage and never entertained the possibility of losing. They had a job to do: deliver the message that a new kingdom was about to be established in their land. They didn't negotiate. They didn't try to "sell" the benefits of the new kingdom. They didn't try to "market" their kingdom so that the citizens of the new land would like them. They simply announced that a major victory was about to take place and offered these options to the soon-to-be conquered territory: You can be civil, or you can be hostile. You can accept our new kingdom, or you can fight it. Either way, we're gonna win. And they did. It didn't matter whether the enemy fought or surrendered. These four kingdoms gained world dominance by not accepting even the hint of resistance. They knew they had the superior army. They knew the outcome before any battle began.

The fifth world kingdom is the one that God is establishing. If you want to see how it ends, read the book of Revelation. It's confusing to some, but the ending is clear: God wins. Big-time. And it's the *final* world kingdom because it will last for eternity. There will never be another war, and everyone in the kingdom will celebrate forever in the presence of God. As a Christian, you are an ambassador for that kingdom. Not a minor player or an insignificant bystander.

You're an ambassador. Your job is to deliver the message: "God reigns over all. He has already won. How you deal with it is up to you. You can be civil or hostile. It doesn't matter to God, though it will make a big difference for you."

It is in that spirit of strength, power, and courage that God expects you to live. Ambassadors don't go around apologizing for their leader. They are not ashamed of their kingdom's values. And as God's ambassador, you have two things going for you. First, you *know* the kingdom you represent has already won the battle over evil. And second, you know the values of your kingdom give each citizen the best life possible. You're not announcing a kingdom ruled by a despot who could care less about its people. God's laws were not created to make life miserable for you. They are not restrictive, as some would have us believe, but freeing. Can you think of a better kingdom to represent than God's?

Does this mean we should get involved in politics? Absolutely, if politics means fighting for what's right. Whenever people criticize me for encouraging Christians to join the political process, I think of where I would be today if another Christian listened to similar critics of his day—the British politician William Wilberforce. You may already know his story, which inspired a wonderful movie, *Amazing Grace*. Wilberforce began his political career in 1780, and in 1785 he became a Christian, which resulted in a major change in his lifestyle, including a passion for reforming society. From that point on, he campaigned vigorously to eradicate slavery in the British Empire, fighting what many considered to be an unwinnable battle and facing scorn from the media and political establishment. Sound familiar? Finally, after forty-eight years of battle, just three days before Wilberforce died, the British Parliament passed the Slavery Abolition Act in 1833.

(By the way, supporters of slavery argued that African slaves were lesser human beings — the same message I heard when I was growing up in Alabama more than a hundred years later.)

Should Christians get involved in politics? Wilberforce actually asked that question after he became a Christian. At that period in British society, Christians in politics were considered religious zealots and he briefly considered leaving politics because it would expose him to so much contempt and ridicule. He consulted with the former slave trader and fellow Christian John Newton and the future prime minister William Pitt, who convinced him to remain in politics so that he could influence society for the better.

While we remember Wilberforce for his opposition to slavery, his Christian values were evident in other reforms he supported. He pushed to enact laws that led to the reform of England's notoriously inhumane prisons, and he passed measures limiting capital punishment. He campaigned for greater support for the poor and is credited with starting Sunday schools for the poor in his district. He even helped to form the Society for the Prevention of Cruelty to Animals.

In fact, throughout our own history, many of the laws and institutions that reformed society for the better were initiated by people who believed in mixing faith with politics. Our own anti-slavery movement included many prominent politicians who voted against slavery because of their Christian beliefs. The American Sunday school movement was largely an effort to fight child labor laws. Many of our best and most successful hospitals were started by churches in order to care for the medical needs of the poor. If a Christian named William Wilberforce had not fought almost his entire adult life to end slavery, I might still be considered three-fifths human in this country, and you might be sitting in your segregated churches feeling good about yourselves.

So why shouldn't *you* step up to the plate and use whatever means you have to fight for what's right? How fortunate we are to live in a country where we have a voice! What can possibly be gained by remaining silent in the face of evil? What hope can you or anyone else have of a better life if you stand idly by and let conditions deteriorate? This quote, often attributed to the Irish statesman, Edmund Burke, still speaks truth: "All that is necessary for evil to triumph is for good men to do nothing." Imagine if everyone who loves God decided to do *something*—voting against a referendum, writing a letter to an elected official, showing up at a Right to Life rally, or anything else that announces the kingdom of God.

As an ambassador of that kingdom, you don't have to be timid about your beliefs. You can represent God's kingdom with power, strength, and courage. Because you know the end of the story, you can ignore all the whiners and complainers who try to convince you it's impossible to stand up for what's right. You've been given a message: the kingdom of God is at hand. It's coming, and there's nothing you can do about it. Civil or hostile. It doesn't matter.

To the rest of the world, you might look like an underdog. Your neighbor might laugh at you when you ask him to sign a petition against a proposal that will allow his teenaged daughter to have an abortion without his consent or awareness. The people you work with might roll their eyes when they hear that you believe God has ordained marriage to be between a man and a woman. The sophisticated pundits might try to paint you the same way they painted Wilberforce — as a religious fanatic. And you might hear your views made fun of on some late-night TV show.

So what? What are you afraid of? What power do they have over you? There is absolutely nothing that can separate you from God's love. There is absolutely no force — political or otherwise — that will triumph over God's plan for his kingdom.

When all is said and done, guess who's going to be celebrating in the locker room? God has a victory party waiting for you that you're not going to believe.

And it's going to last forever.

How Long Is Forever?

A little boy sat on the side of his hospital bed, waiting for the nurse to come to take him for his treatment. Diagnosed with leukemia just three weeks ago, he had already been poked and prodded enough by doctors and nurses to begin to feel at home in the hospital. Although he was only eleven years old, he was smart enough to know he had a serious disease. His parents did their best to shield him from the doctor's prognosis, but he knew. Kids who got his form of leukemia seldom lived more than two years after it was discovered. He could sense that his mom didn't want to talk about it, but her reluctance didn't stop him.

"Mom, I'm gonna die, aren't I?" he asked in a matter-of-fact voice as his mom sat in a chair opposite his bed. The sun shone brightly through the window, and the muffled sound of the traffic outside mingled with the clanging of lunch trays being slid into the big cart in the hallway.

"Why, Timmy, we don't know that for sure." She didn't consider it a lie, rationalizing to herself that although the doctors gave him only six to nine months, everyone at church was praying for a miracle. *Who knows for sure? Maybe God will spare him*, she thought to herself.

"It's OK, Mom. You can tell me the truth. I'm a big boy."

That's when she started to cry. She couldn't help herself. It was just too much for her to handle, knowing not only that her son had so little time but that he also would likely suffer from the treatments. She looked away, not wanting her tears to upset Timmy.

"Don't worry, Mom," he answered in his familiar sing-song voice. "I'm not really going to die."

"That's more like it, Timmy," she smiled as she dabbed a tissue at her damp eyes. "Besides, right now you need to think of how the medicine they're going to give you will race through your body and zap all those bad cells." She managed a chuckle, hoping to take Timmy's mind off the thought of dying.

"No, really Mom. When Uncle Norm visited me, he told me I was going to live forever and that it will only seem like seconds before I get to see you and Dad and Becky again."

She lowered her eyes briefly and thought to herself, *Oh, I hope that's true. I really do.*

Just Passing Through

No wonder they say "out of the mouths of children"

to refer to the wisdom of kids like Timmy. He gets it. His uncle Norm taught him well and gave him a wonderful gift that put his sickness into perspective. Several years ago, Dr. Diane Komp, a highly respected pediatric oncologist who specialized in a particularly deadly disease that afflicts children, wrote a book called *A Child Shall Lead Them*. She explains how she came to faith in God by watching her young patients die. Most people have the exact opposite reaction: the death of innocent children drives them away from believing in a loving and compassionate God. But Dr. Komp was greatly impressed by the children who faced death with the childlike belief that they would go to heaven. They even comforted their parents with this assurance that what awaited them was better than what they were leaving.

That's the kind of hope Tyler Doughtie had, and it was so contagious that even an embittered mailman was drawn to it.

There is nothing childish about Timmy's childlike perspective, because it comes straight from God's Word. The Bible makes it clear that we will live forever, either in heaven with God or in hell separated from God. Forever. Do you have any idea how long forever is? The human mind really can't comprehend *forever*. Forever to many of us is how long we have to wait for our order at McDonald's. We measure time in terms of our lifetime here on earth. For most people, that's anywhere from seventy-five to eighty-five years. God measures time in terms of eternity. I once heard someone try to explain what eternity is compared to our time on earth. He said if you made a dot on a piece of paper and then drew a line across the page and kept extending that line across a million pages, you can begin to understand what eternity is all about. That dot represented your time on this earth, while the line represents eternity. That's a pretty good try, but it falls way short because, in reality, that line a million pages long represents closer to just *one second* in eternity.

To put it in the simplest of terms, however long you live in this world, you're going to live at least a million times longer in the next. And the *way* you live in this world is preparing you for your life in the next.

Jesus tried to get this point across to people by telling a story parable about a rich man and a poor beggar. He understood that the concepts of eternity and of heaven and hell were difficult for our mortal minds to grasp, so he put it in terms that were more familiar.

> There was a rich man who was dressed in purple and fine linen and lived in luxury every day. At his gate was laid a beggar named Lazarus, covered with sores and longing to eat what fell from the rich man's table. Even the dogs came and licked his sores.
>
> Luke 16:19–21

Lazarus (not the Lazarus whom Jesus brought back from the dead) eventually died and went to heaven. The rich man also died, and because he had rejected Jesus, he was sent to hell. He was so tormented by the conditions in hell that when he looked up and saw the Old Testament patriarch Abraham, he asked him to dip his finger in water "and cool my tongue, because I am in agony in this fire" (Luke 16:24). Abraham told him he couldn't fulfill this request because while Lazarus was still living on earth, he had lived only to please himself. He had made a choice and now had to live with it forever. And furthermore, Abraham told him there was a wide chasm separating them. Those in heaven can never cross over into hell, while those in hell can never cross over into heaven.

The rich man had chosen to live his life as if it was the only life he had to live. He made sure he grabbed all the gusto he could while he still had time, with little thought of what was going to happen when he died. The poor man had accepted God's generous offer of salvation, so despite the fact that he was a lowly beggar who had suffered while on earth, he was enjoying an eternal reward in heaven. One man had a few years of living high on the hog followed by an eternity of despair; the other man had a few years of poverty followed by an eternity in the presence of God.

Who Would You Rather Be?

Back in the day, we used to sing a chorus that began,

"This world is not my home, I'm just passing through." It echoes the teaching of the apostle Peter, who describes Christians as "aliens and strangers in the world" (1 Peter 2:11). Aliens and strangers don't belong, and as citizens of God's final kingdom, our home on earth is only a temporary residence. One of the reasons so many people live such unhappy lives is that they think what we have now is all there is. They have grown too comfortable with their temporary homes here on earth, forgetting that they have a better home that will last forever. So they chase after things they think will satisfy them because they don't want to miss out on a good time, repeating the process over and over until they reach the end and wonder where the years went. What they don't realize is that if they live the way God wants them to, life on earth will give them true satisfaction, and they will have the rest of eternity to enjoy not just a good time but the best.

What Heaven Does for You Today

You've heard the phrase "Some people are so heavenly minded that they are no earthly good" (often attributed to Oliver Wendell Holmes). It's usually aimed at people like me who actually believe in heaven. But as far as I'm concerned, you can't be too heavenly minded. We are told by Saint Paul, "Since, then, you have been raised with Christ, set your hearts on things above, where Christ is seated at the right hand of God. Set your minds on things above, not on earthly things" (Colossians 3:1–2). In fact, our problem is that we don't think about heaven enough. It's *because* I believe in heaven that I want to do as much as I can while I'm here, knowing, as I do, that the time is so short.

Focusing on heaven helps us keep our priorities straight. Just because I'm looking forward to an eternal party with God and all the other people who will join me in heaven doesn't mean I've given up on life here on earth. Why do you think I've become such a pain in the behind to anyone who tries to legalize things the Bible considers immoral? I'm doing my best while I'm here to make the world a better place. As Christians, that's our assignment. My church doesn't even own a building so that we can have more money to help people rebuild their lives and become productive citizens. Just because a person believes in heaven doesn't give him or her a free pass to sit around and wait for it. The great Christian writer C. S. Lewis stated, "If you read history you will find that the Christians who did most for the present world were just those who thought most of the next.... It is since Christians have largely ceased to think of the other world that they have become so ineffective in this."* I'm looking forward to being able to take it easy and enjoy myself for the rest of eternity, but while I'm here, I want to make the best of it. God has never given up on his earthly kingdom, and he expects his followers to do

*C. S. Lewis, *Mere Christianity* (anniversary ed.; New York: Macmillan, 1981), 113.

whatever they can to redeem and restore it. We will never make a "heaven on earth," but that reality should never stop us from trying because it prepares us for the true heaven.

Believing in heaven puts everything in proper perspective. It makes living here worry free, because whatever happens here and now not only has a purpose but is a brief prelude to forever. Shortly before he was arrested, Jesus sensed that his disciples were worried. He had just told them that he knew he would soon be killed, and they simply could not imagine life without him. He comforted them with heaven, which he described as his Father's house with "many mansions" (John 14:2 KJV). He explained that he was leaving them so that he could go and prepare a mansion for every one of them and that he would return and take them back with him into their new eternal homes. It is that knowledge that encouraged his followers to do God's work on earth and sustained a movement that today stretches around the world.

The poor beggar who waited for crumbs from the rich man's table knew that even if the rich man invited him inside for dinner, an entire banquet was waiting for him in heaven. Having no money and being covered with sores was nothing compared to what was in store for him. Whenever I'm experiencing a lot of pain from my disease and beginning to feel down when I think I might not be around to see my daughters get married, I remind myself that a few days of pain is a small price to pay to become more like Jesus.

And a few days is such a short time when compared to a forever of perfect peace and joy. The instant my heart stops beating, I will be incapable of feeling sad about anything. And in what will seem like yet another instant — literally the blink of an eye — my daughters and their husbands, my grandkids, my sons and their wives, my wife, Pat, and everyone else I love will join me in a great reunion. And we'll have plenty of time to get caught up on things. I actually get excited thinking about it.

Knowing that we have an eternity ahead of us that is perfect in all its aspects gives us the motivation and courage to do the things we know we need to do in order to experience the best in life. It's like an Olympic swimmer who has to get in the pool every day to train. Every morning she wakes up and is tempted to roll over and stay in bed. Skip today's workout. But instead she swings one leg out of bed and then the other and leaves the warmth and comfort of her bed, heads for the pool, and jumps in. Lap after lap she pushes herself to the limit, gasping for air as she recovers, only to repeat the drill again and again. And when the coach whistles the end of her workout, she voluntarily grinds out a few extra laps. Why would anyone subject themselves to such pain? Because she pictures herself standing on the awards stand at the Olympic Games, bending slightly as the official places the gold medal around her neck and her nation's anthem plays over the loudspeakers. The hope of earning that medal kept her going in that pool, far away from the spotlight. If you interviewed that champion and asked her about all those mornings in the pool, she would probably say, "Compared to this medal around my neck, it was nothing!"

Heaven gives you that same hope. It motivates you to do the right thing—to get up every morning, jump into your day, and live like a champion. Even though your future in heaven was secured the moment you became a Christian, you continue to be faithful because you know what awaits you there—and it's a lot better than a gold medal.

David Livingstone was a Scottish missionary to Africa in the nineteenth century. One of the reasons he chose Africa is that he wanted to abolish the slave trade, and he felt that by opening up missions stations all across Africa it would deter traders (thank you, Dr. Livingstone!). To get the job done he became the first European to cross the entire African continent. But it came at a cost. On one of his first journeys deep into Africa to set up a mission post, he was mauled by a tiger. The resulting injury plagued him with pain for the rest of his life. At various times he also suffered from malaria and dysentery, and in fact he died in Africa of malaria. On a trip back to England to recruit more missionaries he spoke about his "sacrifice" to take the gospel to Africa:

> People talk of the sacrifice I have made in spending so much of my life in Africa. Can that be called a sacrifice which is simply paid back as a small part

of a great debt owing to our God, which we can never repay? Is that a sacrifice which brings its own blest reward in healthful activity, the consciousness of doing good, peace of mind, and a bright hope of a glorious destiny hereafter? Away with the word in such a view, and with such a thought! It is emphatically no sacrifice. Say rather it is a privilege. Anxiety, sickness, suffering, or danger, now and then, with a foregoing of the common conveniences and charities of this life, may make us pause, and cause the spirit to waver, and the soul to sink, but let this only be for a moment. All these are nothing when compared with the glory which shall hereafter be revealed in and for us. I never made a sacrifice.*

Dr. Livingstone knew that his eternal home was waiting for him. Any temptation to quit and go back to Scotland left him when he remembered where he was going.

On the other hand, if you're not heavenly minded, all you have to motivate you to do the things you ought to be doing—the things you really want to do—is your own willpower. That works—some of the time. But eventually you lose heart and fall back into your old ways. That's why good, decent church folk have such a hard time fighting the battles we are called to fight. They begin with good

*Quoted in William Garden Blaikie, *The Personal Life of David Livingstone* (New York: Revell, 1880), 243 (from a lecture to students at Cambridge University, December 4, 1857).

intentions but soon grow weary and retreat into the comfort of their own little worlds. Once you understand and truly believe in the reality of heaven, you won't think twice about jumping into that pool like the Olympic swimmer and training for your reward. The great revival preacher of the nineteenth century, Charles Spurgeon, put it this way when he spoke about heaven: "To come to thee is to come home from exile, to come to land out of the raging storm, to come to rest after long labor, to come to the goal of my desires and the summit of my wishes."*

Believing in heaven gives focus to your life on earth. It sets your heart on the things that matter, deflecting those distractions that can prevent you from living the life you truly desire. Martin Luther once wrote that as far as he was concerned, only two days were important: today and the day he enters heaven. In other words, we don't have to worry about tomorrow because our future is certain. Knowing this truth liberates us to do whatever God wants us to do today, regardless of the cost. As Christians, we are to live as if today is the last day we have on earth. If you live that way, your job as an ambassador takes on a certain urgency. Who needs to hear today that the kingdom of God is coming? Who needs to be given the good news so that they, too, can join you in heaven?

Finally, heaven erases your fear of dying. Guess what?

---

*Charles Spurgeon, *Morning by Morning* (New York: Sheldon, 1867), 116.

The current death rate is 100 percent. Always has been. Always will be. Ten out of ten people will die. Death is inevitable; no one escapes it, and for most people it is one of their greatest fears. Look at the lengths we have gone to in order to extend our lives. As recently as the 1930s the average life span was barely more than fifty years; now it's more than seventy-five years. I'm thankful for all the advances in science and medicine that have extended our lives. Even now, having a disease that should have killed me years ago, I'm thrilled to still be alive. It's normal and natural to want to live. But knowing that I will have an even better life after I die takes the fear out of dying. Talk about contagious hope!

I've gotten to know the medical folks who take care of me when I get really sick, and they know the score when it comes to my chances. When they learn that I have absolutely no fear of dying, they want to know more. So I tell them, and just because of my hope in heaven, there are going to be a lot more people with lab coats and stethoscopes joining me there! In fact, I think I know why God hasn't taken me home yet. I've had a couple of wonderful doctors who have cared for me — among the best in the nation. I have come to love them, and I pray every day that they will accept God's free gift of salvation. And I'm doing everything I can to show them just how great it is to be loved by God. I just have this feeling that God is using me to be a positive witness for him with these two doctors.

It's not that he needs me, because he could use anyone if I wasn't around. But for whatever reason, he gave me an assignment that's part of his grand plan of redemption, so he's keeping me going until I complete my assignment.

The Rest of the Story

A lot of people would like me to end right there. Give people a little taste of heaven, and leave it at that. Hold out the hope of heaven, and let people think they've got a chance. Everybody likes the idea of heaven, and a lot of people think that's where we'll all end up. But the truth is, not everyone will go to heaven. Only those who have received God's gift of salvation will go to heaven. The rest go somewhere else. The place we don't like to talk about — hell.

I *wish* everyone could go to heaven. I really do. And I'm doing all I can to make sure as many people as I can influence will join me there. The reason I do so is because I don't want anyone to suffer in hell. And the Bible makes it very clear that those who reject Jesus will be banished to hell. Forever. Just as those who believe in Christ will spend eternity with him in heaven, those who reject him will spend eternity separated from him in hell.

I know this isn't the most popular teaching in the Bible. There was a time early in our nation's history when pretty much everyone believed in hell. But as we have become more and more secularized, the concept of hell has been rejected, and people like me who believe in it are considered foolish and unsophisticated. Sadly, even a lot of preachers act as if they don't believe in hell. They either deny its existence outright or try to explain it away with human logic. A good and loving God would never make anyone suffer forever. You make your own hell on earth — it doesn't really exist anywhere else. You don't really suffer punishment forever but are vaporized and simply cease to exist. Some even teach that everyone eventually gets to heaven.

The only source of what I believe is the Bible, and if anyone can show me where the Bible teaches any of these things about hell, I'll change my beliefs. Jesus warns us of the Enemy, Satan, "who can destroy both soul and body in hell" (Matthew 10:28). He teaches that if any part of your body causes you to sin, it would be better to lose it "than for your whole body to be thrown into hell" (Matthew 5:29). He compares those who reject his salvation to weeds that will be pulled from the ground and thrown into "the fiery furnace, where there will be weeping and gnashing of teeth" (Matthew 13:42).

No one really knows for sure what hell is like, but from the Bible's description it is clear that it will be severe. It will include physical pain, the type that is associated with fire. Have you ever burned yourself? Imagine that pain over your entire body. When you burn your finger, the pain is intense, but it is usually gone within a day or two. The physical pain of hell lasts forever.

But the physical pain will be nothing compared to the emotional pain of separation from God, family, and friends. Have you ever been homesick or lonely? I have. I hate to be away from my family, but what keeps me going is knowing I will eventually get to see them again. In hell, the loneliness is permanent. Eternal.

But it goes deeper. Have you ever felt that God had abandoned you? That he wasn't listening to your prayers or had turned his back on you? Of course, he hasn't, but in our human frailty, sometimes it seems as if God has forgotten about us when our prayers aren't answered or when bad things happen to us. But in hell, it's for real. He *has* abandoned you, and you will be separated from him forever.

"Hutch, why'd you have to go there? I thought this was a book about hope."

If you took your family on a vacation in the mountains and hiked a trail that eventually led to the edge of a steep cliff, would you warn your children about the cliff ahead, or would you let them run in front of you and discover it themselves? Millions of people are racing toward something far worse than a cliff, and it's our job as Christians to warn them. If they continue the race without accepting Jesus as their Savior, their lives are hopeless. But if they know what lies ahead at the end of their brief lives on earth, they can make a choice that will give them lasting hope.

Earlier I wrote that if everyone could spend twenty-four hours in hell, they would all go to heaven. Actually, twenty-four *seconds* would be enough to convince them they would never want to return. I know of a man who had just finished mowing the lawn, and his toddler son wandered over to the mower and reached out to touch it. Knowing that the hot engine would burn his son, the dad grabbed his little boy's hand and attempted to place it just close enough to the engine so that he could feel the heat. Unfortunately, he accidentally brushed his son's little hand onto the engine for the briefest of seconds, but it was enough to cause the boy to shriek in pain and to have a nasty blister pop up on his hand. Of course, the dad felt horrible about burning his son's finger by mistake, but he also reported that from that point on, his son never went near the lawn mower.

That's why I have to tell you the rest of the story about our eternal lives. The Bible says that Christ does not want *anyone* to perish (2 Peter 3:9). He has provided a way for you and me to avoid spending an eternity in hell. Our privilege as Christians is to offer this hope to everyone we meet. I love to preach about heaven, but I can't ignore the alternative. And neither can you.

Some Arrive Early

I can't explain why a little child like Timmy had to die so young. What I know with absolute certainty is that for those who accept Jesus as their Savior, it's all good because the trials we face make us more and more like Jesus. I also know that God sees things we will never see, and perhaps he saw a future ahead of Timmy that would give him more pain than he could bear. The Bible teaches that God comes to help us and will not allow any of his followers to endure more than they can handle (1 Corinthians 10:13). Perhaps taking Timmy home early was a way to fulfill that promise.

Because of heaven, I also know that Timmy is having the time of his life. Because of heaven, I have all the hope I need to live well in my temporary home.

And so do you.

Shine like a Superstar

Of all the weddings I've presided over as a minister, I've never seen an ugly bride.

That doesn't mean every woman who got married in my church was beautiful. Some were, but just as many were rather ordinary in their appearance. A few have been overweight. I need to be careful here because my church folk will be reading this book, and I don't want someone coming up to me and asking, "Was that me you were writing about?" But maybe one or two of the women from all of those weddings I've performed might be considered, um— how should I say this?—interesting.

Be careful, Hutch.

But I've never seen an ugly bride. Something happens when a woman walks down the aisle to meet her man and pledge her love to him. She *becomes* beautiful. You see her before the wedding, and she's quite average, but when she stands in front of me with her man, she's so beautiful it makes old men wish they were young again. You know what I'm talking about. You go to a wedding, take your seat, and wait as a couple of cute kids struggle to light the candles. Then the attendants march to the front, and if one of them is your daughter, you just beam because she's clearly the most beautiful girl in the church, next to your wife. Then there's that signal from the organist, and we all rise to our feet and face the back of the church. And what you see almost takes your breath away. The most beautiful woman in the world slowly makes her way to the front. I'm not sayin' it's a miracle, but something happened to that woman. Maybe it's the dress or the fancy work done by her hairdresser or the makeup. Or maybe it really is a miracle, but I've never seen an ugly bride.

Can't always say the same for the groom. You can dress some guy up in the fanciest tuxedo around, and he's *still* ugly. But not his bride. You can almost see it in his eyes: *How did such an ugly guy like me get such a beautiful woman?* I can't explain it. It's just the way it is.

The Bible uses an amazing phrase to describe the church: *the bride of Christ.* It's a beautiful image that explains the relationship between Jesus and all who call him Savior. Figuratively, we are wedded to him, only this marriage will last forever. At present, we are physically separated from Jesus, but we are promised that one day he will return to claim his bride. As believers, we wait with great anticipation for that to happen. One of the reasons there are no ugly brides is that as the wedding day approaches, brides get ready. I mean they really get ready. My girls haven't gotten married yet, mostly because I won't allow it until they are thirty-five! But some of my buddies who've been through it tell me to start saving. First it's the gown, then just the right shoes, then a new wardrobe for the honeymoon. As the date approaches, add in a manicure and a pedicure. Then that trip to the hairstylist. That's just for *her*. The church will be elaborately decorated with flowers and candles. All of her attendants will wear matching gowns and carry bouquets of flowers.

All you dads who have ever paid for a wedding—your daughters don't do this to spite you. They want everything to be perfect. Beautiful. Because it's their wedding, and they are the bride. Every bride wants her groom to stand at the altar with anticipation and be completely smitten by his beautiful bride.

So when Jesus returns to greet you, what kind of bride will he see? Will she be ugly, or will she be beautiful?

What Be Your Attitude?

Up to this point, we've been looking at how and why you can have hope. We've been seeing that real hope can only come when you recognize God's sovereignty—that this hope enables you to face "all things" gladly because you know it is making you more like Jesus. And we've discovered how you can hope to live the life you really want to live because of God's Holy Spirit at work in you.

But if you think God wants you to have hope for *your* sake, you're making that age-old mistake of thinking it's all about you. It's not. If you think that this hope is only about getting to heaven, then all you've got is fire insurance. The hope God gives you is part of his great and generous plan to redeem his world. He has given you this hope so that you will stand out from the crowd. He knows how desperately people need hope, and the best way for them to find it is to see it reflected from you. Like the bride who has been so transformed that it takes our breath away, the hope that you have been given should have the same effect on everyone who comes into contact with you.

I've preached more than a thousand sermons in my life, but Jesus preached only one — at least there's only one recorded in the Bible. He obviously preached more, but his Sermon on the Mount is the only one whose complete text was preserved for us. Sermons are generally meant for Christians, and in this case, Jesus was indeed preaching to Christ-followers who had gathered on the gently sloping hills near the Sea of Galilee. Nothing in the Bible is there by accident, so if this is the only sermon written down for us to read, it's got to be important.

Although this event occurred at the beginning of Jesus' ministry on earth, he knew that eventually the church would be continuing his work of proclaiming the Good

News of salvation through him. Many scholars who have studied this sermon consider it to be an instruction book for how Christians are to live. Once Jesus moves past the introduction, he deals with everything from adultery to fasting. But in the opening section of the sermon, he teaches us how to turn our hope into something that's contagious. He shows us how to make sure his bride is so beautiful that others are drawn to her. These verses are often referred to as the Beatitudes (Matthew 5:3 – 12), which means "blessedness" or "bliss." Jesus knew that no matter how much we invite others to join his kingdom, the wrong attitude can turn people away. So he repeats nine times the attitude we must have if we are to be his beautiful bride — an attitude of blessedness.

"That's it, Hutch? *Blessedness?*"

I preached on this once in my church, and I got the same reaction. Only other preachers will recognize the look: heads nodding up and down, faces frozen in bewilderment. They're trying to be polite and act as if you just said something important, but I could tell. They weren't buying it. And I immediately knew why. They didn't have a clue what *blessedness* meant. Probably their only context for the word has to do with sneezing ("Bless you!"). So I'm up there preaching my heart out, and they're wondering why I'm getting all excited about sneezes.

Blessedness is one of those words like *glory*. It sounds morbidly religious. Boring. Old ladies pat little kids on the head and say, "Bless your heart." Some people say a blessing before they eat. It's not a bad word, but to most people it's plain vanilla. Tame. Until they understand what it means.

Some well-meaning people have translated the word *blessed* as "happy," but that's a poor translation. Happy is often superficial. Happy comes and goes. You can be happy one moment and unhappy the next. And in some cases, happy is inappropriate. God doesn't expect you to be happy when your house burns down. A better word for blessedness is *joy*. Or as the *NIV Study Bible* puts it, " 'Blessed' here refers to the ultimate well-being and distinctive spiritual joy of those who share in the salvation of the kingdom of God." As I've said throughout this book, God wants to give you the best. Ultimate is the best. It doesn't get any better than ultimate. That's what blessedness is—the ultimate in satisfaction, peace, and joy.

So Jesus is preaching to a group of Christ-followers, knowing that in addition to the normal misfortunes they would face in life, they would also be persecuted for their faith. So he lists some of the things he knew would interrupt their lives. In each situation, he describes the attitude they should have:

> If you are poor in spirit, discouraged, downtrodden, finding that things aren't going your way—you *are* blessed, filled with the ultimate in joy and satisfaction.
>
> If you mourn or are genuinely sad about something—you *are* blessed.

> If you are meek, humble, not very important in the eyes of others — you *are* blessed.
>
> If you desperately want to do the right thing, regardless of what everyone else does — you *are* blessed.
>
> If you show mercy and compassion to others in a self-centered world — you *are* blessed.
>
> If you remain pure in your thoughts and actions in a world that revels in impurity — you *are* blessed.
>
> If you bring peace when you are surrounded by turmoil and fighting — you *are* blessed.
>
> If you are persecuted because you live the way I have instructed you — you *are* blessed.
>
> If people make fun of you or spread rumors about you or accuse you of being narrow-minded because you identify with me — you *are* blessed.

Verbs are important in the Bible, which is why I put this helping verb in italics. Jesus didn't say if you face all of these things you *will* be blessed. The joy and ultimate well-being for those who share in the salvation of God won't be yours *someday*; they are yours *right now*, as you are going through these things. Of course you're going to face things that are unpleasant when you follow Jesus, and they might not make you happy. But you can experience something better than happiness. The problem with most of us is that we think we have to be happy all the time, and since it's impossible to be happy when we're going through the fire, we fake it, and that's why so many people think Christians are phony. You can't fake joy. And you can't hide it either. It's what you see in the face of a true follower of Christ who is out of work. He's not happy, but he has that ultimate sense of well-being because he knows that God is in control and that whatever the effects of unemployment may be, they can't compare to being molded into the very image of Jesus. There's a children's chorus that comes straight from Scripture that illustrates this: "The joy of the Lord is my strength." That's what Jesus was preaching on that mountain. Forget happiness. I've got something better. What I've got for you lasts for every step you take on this difficult journey.

Keep Your Mirror Polished

Like everything else God gives you, this gift of joy isn't just for you or even *about* you. Certainly, you benefit from this attitude that he has given you. Ask anyone who has gone through something difficult and has experienced this ultimate sense of well-being — this peace that expresses itself as joy. A few years ago, a family lost one of their daughters in a tragic accident in Indiana. A student at a Christian college, this young woman was known for her strong faith in God, which she learned as a child from her parents. These were godly people who served the Lord in their church — real "salt of the earth" people who were well-known in their community. One of the television reporters covering the story remarked about how well the parents seemed to be handling this awful loss. I don't recall the exact quote, but it went something like this: "Of course they are sad, but they just seem to be so at peace with it." In fact, their "ultimate sense of well-being" was so contagious that their story was told in a best-selling book (*Mistaken Identity*).

And now we can see the real reason Jesus asks us to accept this attitude of joy. As much as it benefits us by giving us the strength to endure anything, the real benefit is to his kingdom—his plan to redeem to himself as many as possible. Shortly after introducing his sermon with these beatitudes, he declares, "You are the light of the world" (Matthew 5:14). If you were to ask most people who the light of the world is, they would say Jesus, and they would be right. Jesus says as much in the book of John: "I am the light of the world" (John 8:12). So when he tells us that *we* are the light of the world, he means we are to reflect *his* light. We are to be mirrors of his radiant light so that it attracts others to him. The joy and ultimate sense of well-being that is to be our attitude is really his attitude. When you get a flat tire on the way to work, and it's raining and you arrive at your job a half hour late, soaked and grumpy, you have an opportunity to hold your mirror up to Jesus and to let your coworkers see his joy, his peace, his truth that everything has a purpose and that it's good. Or you can stomp through the building to your work station, cursing your luck, whining and complaining about the weather, and getting as much pity as you can from your colleagues. What kind of person do you want to be? Who do you want to reflect to those who know you go to church and occasionally try to get your colleagues to accept your Jesus?

Christians, especially those who go by the adjective *evangelical*, know they have been given a mission: to invite others into a relationship with Jesus. For the most part, we do it quite well. We have developed elaborate plans to help us share our faith. We have learned how to proclaim the gospel by means of little diagrams and illustrations. We sponsor seminars and conferences to teach people how to talk to their friends about Jesus. And we can choose from dozens of excellent books that show us how to effectively tell others about God's free gift of salvation. In my church, sharing our faith is one of our top priorities. But we can have all the right words and yet have the wrong attitude — and we're going to do more harm than good. Jesus knew that people who are hungry for fulfillment will watch what we do more than listen to what we say. He knew we would be tested, but he gave us the perfect resource — one that makes our own lives better as it leads people to his truth. He gave us a mirror. It's as though we hear him saying, "Just aim that mirror on me and let my light shine, and everything's going to be all right."

Don't Build Your Own Fire

Some well-intentioned Christians read that they are the light of the world and get a big head. They get the light part but forget where it comes from. They go to church every Sunday and carry their Bibles to work with them. They volunteer at the homeless shelter and make sure all their friends know about it. When their friends invite them to go to the casino, they politely refuse: "I don't gamble; it's a bad habit, you know." Nothing wrong with all the good things they do, but they're making sure the light is shining on *them*. They dropped their mirrors and began building their own little fires. That's why so many people think Christians are holier-than-thou. They're smart enough to know all that stuff is for show. Sometimes even the little things we do that we think are right give off the wrong attitude. Have you ever seen that bumper sticker that reads, "I'm not perfect, just forgiven." It's absolutely true, but it can come off as arrogant. It's like saying, "I'm forgiven, and you're not." It puts the spotlight on you. Maybe they should change the message to read, "I'm not perfect, but God is." That reflects *his* light, not our own.

Jesus knew how easy it would be for us to begin to take credit for the good things we do. When he gets into the meat of his sermon (Matthew 6:1 – 18), he warns against shining the light on ourselves.

> When you help out the poor, don't make a big deal about it; instead, do these deeds of compassion in secret, where only God can see your generosity.
> Don't be like the hypocrites who recite ornate prayers

in public so everyone can see how spiritual they are;
instead, go into a room by yourself and pray.

If you decide to fast, don't go around looking all hungry
and sad; instead, smile and say nothing about it to
anyone.

Have you ever been around someone who gives up
something for Lent? All she can talk about is how horrible
it is to go without coffee or chocolate for forty days. The
actual purpose for this tradition during Lent is to experience a suffering that calls us to remember the suffering of
Jesus, not to make ourselves look religious. But oh my, hang
out with someone who can't have her roast beef, and you'd
think Lent was all about her.

Even in Old Testament times before Jesus appeared,
God understood our tendency to think that everything
revolves around us. He knew that whenever anything good
happens to us, we are quick to take the credit. It's that age-
old struggle with sovereignty. Who's really in charge? In
the book of Isaiah God warns us about trying to be the
light rather than reflect the light, and he uses the image of
fire. "Walk in the light of your fires and of the torches you
have set ablaze," and here's what you get from me: "You will
lie down in torment" (Isaiah 50:11). Would God give you
such a smackdown for doing all the right things? If you do it
without reflecting the true light, you can bet on it. If you're
trying to be the light of the world and things aren't going

well for you, maybe you should check to see whose light you're reflecting, yours or God's.

Twinkle, Twinkle

Wherever Jesus went, crowds came out to see him. Hundreds, even thousands, of people dropped what they were doing and rushed to meet him. We seldom see him alone—only when he went into the wilderness to wrestle with the Enemy, when he pushed out into the middle of the lake to escape the crowds and test Peter's water wings, and finally in a garden on the night of his arrest when he knew a cruel death was coming and asked God if he really had to go through with it. The rest of the time he was surrounded by people. Men and women. Old and young. Jews and Gentiles. They were all drawn to him because he was a bright light in their dark world. Even when he spoke no words, they were attracted to his demeanor, his attitude. He embodied blessedness—that sense of ultimate well-being. Joy. The light of his very presence was irresistible. If you've ever been lost in the woods at night, there is no more welcome sight than a light. When you see it, you run toward it, relieved that you have found the way out.

Our world is just as dark today as it was when Jesus walked the earth; in fact, I'd venture to say it's even darker. People are confused, frustrated, disillusioned, and angry. Even if they don't know it, they are lost. Alone in a hostile world, trying to find their way out of the mess. In one of his letters to Christians, Saint Paul anticipates what it will be like for Christians to live in a dark world, among a people he describes as a "crooked and depraved generation," so he encourages them to "shine like stars in the universe" (Philippians 2:15). He could have used another image — "blaze like a bonfire" or "glow like a candle." But he used a star instead. Do you remember what led the Magi to Jesus? "We saw his star in the east and have come to worship him" (Matthew 2:2).

Isn't it great to know you can be a star that draws people to Jesus? Doesn't it just overwhelm you with gratitude as you begin to relax and quit trying so hard and just let the King of kings shine through you? When I wrote at the beginning of this book that these years of living with cancer have been the best years of my life, you might have been skeptical. I don't blame you for that attitude. We've been conditioned to think the good life should be free of pain and suffering. Maybe now it's beginning to make sense. My mirror is polished and aimed right at the face of the Savior of the world. When a patient transport associate comes to wheel me into yet another MRI, he doesn't see a black man worried about the results. He may not know it, but he's looking at his only hope. He wouldn't understand the word, but he's seeing someone *blessed*. Someone with a sense of ultimate well-being. Joy. Perfect peace. It's what everybody wants.

"How do you manage so well, Dr. Hutcherson?"

I always smile when they ask this question. It's as

though God is saying to me, "See? I told ya. Stay out of the way. Hold that mirror up, and I'll do the rest. Oh, by the way — see ya later." I almost don't have to answer, but I do.

"It's all Jesus. And it's all good!"

It's All Good!

Football is a violent sport. When a 225-pound running back collides with a 260-pound linebacker, it's equivalent to the impact of an automobile hitting a brick wall at twenty miles per hour, and the passenger isn't wearing a seat belt. Or the impact of a bowling ball dropped to the pavement from the thirteenth floor of a building. On any given play there are at least eleven battles being executed, and the basic strategy is the same for just about all of them: hit or get hit. When I hit those running backs coming through the line or an unfortunate wide receiver running a slant across my territory, I could tell by the funny noises that came out of them that it hurt. I changed my ways some from my high school days when I actually wanted to hurt guys, but not much. It felt good to see your man all wobbly when he got up.

But what a lot of people don't realize, those hits hurt me too. Maybe not as much as it hurt the littler guy, but it still hurt. Maybe my head was in the wrong position when I made a tackle, and I got a stinger in my neck. Or sometimes I'd tackle a guy and end up having his 220-pound body fall on top of me. All those hurts in a game add up. By the time the final seconds ticked off the clock and we headed for the locker room, there's a whole lot of hurtin' goin' on.

There's something funny about those hurts, though. If you lose the game, you seem to ache for days, making it hard to get ready for the next game. You're sitting there in front of your locker and can't even take off your pads because you hurt so much. But in the wining locker room, you hardly feel them. It's like a supernatural healing. You could have sworn you took a knee to the ribs so hard you could hear the crunch of bones snapping, but after a win, the pain seems to have disappeared. And if it's a really big game in which you were the underdog or you were playing for a league championship, you can have a broken foot and you'll be up jumpin' around and high-fivin' like everybody else.

Nothing takes the hurt out of your body like a victory.

Some People Don't Like You

Religious people don't always like to think about it this way, but life is a battle between good and evil. It began before human history when an angel challenged God and was thrown out of heaven and banished forever from his presence. And it will end after Jesus returns to greet his bride — you and me — and God's kingdom will be established forever. As you might guess, I have my views on how everything will play out, but these aren't as important as the outcome: *we win.*

Like any battle, we all take some hits along the way. The early Christians knew what big hits are like. The Romans made a sport out of feeding them to the lions. And throughout history — including current history — Christians have been ridiculed, persecuted, and martyred for their beliefs. If you don't think we're in a battle, consider some of the things we've had to deal with in my brief lifetime. I began my journey as a Christian because my public school allowed Campus Crusade for Christ to sponsor an assembly at which the gospel was presented. Today, most high schools will not allow an invocation to be given at their graduation ceremonies. Despite the fact that some of the best and most highly treasured choral music deals with sacred themes from the Bible, many schools will not allow their music departments to perform these classical numbers. Federal courts have allowed the observance of the African-American holiday called *Kwanzaa* but prohibit schools from celebrating Christmas as a religious holiday. In some public schools, Muslim students are allowed to observe their five-times-a-day prayer time, and if they miss a test because of it, they are allowed to take it later. Can you imagine a Christian student being excused from a test because he wants to pray?

When I was a kid, Lucy and Ricky Ricardo could not be shown sleeping in the same bed, despite the fact that they were married. Can you say *Desperate Housewives?* Whether it's television, movies, or "shock jock" radio, Christian values, which are embraced by the majority of Americans, are not only held up to scorn but have been replaced with an immoral, "anything goes" climate that our grandparents could never have imagined. When I talk about this issue, even many Christians try to tell me it's only business—that there is no deliberate effort by the entertainment industry to influence morality. They're just giving us what we want. Hollywood would create more movies that would appeal to the 100 million Americans who go to church every Sunday if more people would go to them. Oh, really? The highest grossing R-rated movie of all time was an accurate depiction of the final days of Jesus' ministry, *The Passion of the Christ*, but producer Mel Gibson couldn't find a studio to make it and had to put up his own money.

Over the years I've observed that you can take a public stand for anything except your faith. You can protest against the dredging of a river to protect a frog, you can criticize people who wear fur coats, you can protest against circuses because they make tigers jump through hoops, you can protest against oil companies for drilling for oil, and you can protest against farmers because you built a house next to their farm and you don't like the smell. As a citizen of a democracy, I'm all for free speech and the freedom to take a stand for what you believe. So why are Christians considered narrow-minded and intolerant if we take a stand for what we believe?

If you don't think we're in a battle, just ask Francis Collins, one of America's most respected scientists, who headed up the Human Genome Project, which mapped the entire genetic code of the human body. Dr. Collins is also a devout Christian who has spent time debating atheists about the existence of God and speaking about the compatibility of science and Christianity. In the summer of 2009, the president of the United States nominated Dr. Collins to head up the National Institutes of Health. Almost immediately the attacks began from those who do not think a Christian can be a responsible scientist — this despite the fact that Dr. Collins has distinguished himself as a world-renowned geneticist!

If this brief sampling of the battles we face makes you anxious, relax. Remember, it's all good. If you have to experience a little ridicule or criticism for standing up for what's right, there's a purpose behind it. Out here in the Northwest, some people consider me Public Enemy Number One. Big deal. If we're on the winning team, what's to be afraid of? The reason so many of the early Christians sang as they were marched into the coliseum is because they knew the lions couldn't stop them. Likewise, we can live out our faith in the full confidence that we are more than conquerors. If our spiritual ancestors could sing in the face of death, we ought to be able to take a little heat for our beliefs. Nothing can harm us; nothing can stop us. Absolutely nothing. No law. No government. No special interest group. Nothing.

The battle already has been won, so instead of retreating, we ought to act like champions.

One of the things I learned from my high school football coach was to take the field believing we would win. To look like champions. Heading out onto the field with a bit of a swagger. Heads held high, shoulders back. There was just something intimidating about seeing us getting ready for the game that it often took the fight out of our opponents before the game even began. That's good advice for all of us who take the field for God. We don't have to be ashamed about our beliefs. We don't have to apologize for our convictions.

Whenever Christians have been energized and allowed their faith to guide their actions, it has always made things better — from the Constitution's affirmation of the equality of all people to the concept of free education for all citizens to the establishment of the first hospital to the abolition of slavery. When the government couldn't take care of its poor, Christians founded shelters and soup kitchens. The rescue movement for abused and forgotten women that began in the late nineteenth century was started by a church. After abolishing slavery, Christians led the modern civil rights movement that led to laws making it illegal to discriminate against me. The nation's largest nonprofit provider of services for people with disadvantages, Goodwill Industries, was started by a minister.

If you are growing weary in the battle to do right, look around you. Because individual Christians unashamedly let their faith motivate them to get involved — to fight for what was right — millions of people have hope today. We have so much to offer this world — a world that often looks so dark and hopeless. To a world filled with cynicism, we offer trust that the God who is *for* them is in control. To those who despair that life is meaningless, belief gives courage to not just endure but to triumph. To the single mom struggling to raise her teenaged son, we offer a community of nurture and care in the church. To those who see the forces of evil encroaching into their homes, we offer an army led by the Son of God that is willing to stand against immorality. And to those who are tired of the way their lives are going and have discovered that no matter how hard they try they can't find what it is they are looking for, we offer the good news that, regardless of their circumstances, they can have a brand-new life today and an eternity with God in heaven.

Don't Give Up

In Paul's letter to a group of Christians in Galatia, he closes with some practical advice about how to live in a corrupt culture. He warns them of various immoral practices that were prevalent at the time and then lists "the fruit of the Spirit" — character qualities that they ought to have as Christians: "love, joy, peace, patience, kindness, goodness, faithfulness, gentleness and self-control" (Galatians 5:22 – 23). Perhaps realizing that life is hard and messy — and that in an environment that does not honor God it is difficult to stand out in the crowd — he doesn't stop there. He probably knew that whenever individuals try to do the right thing by following God's standards instead of man's, they will be singled out for ridicule and persecution. And from his own experience traveling all over the region as a missionary, being shipwrecked and thrown in prison, he probably also knew how easy it is to get discouraged. So he gives them a little pep talk: "Let us not become weary in doing good, for at the proper time we will reap a harvest if we do not give up" (Galatians 6:9). An old preacher once paraphrased this and had it engraved on index cards for everyone in his church: "Hangeth in there!"

> I know it's not always easy to do what is right. Even though the battle has already been won, the Enemy wants to take as many captives as he can. The forces of darkness often seem insurmountable, and the temptation to retreat to our own little spiritual bunkers is strong. But hang in there.
>
> All the other parents might let their underage kids go to R-rated movies, and your kids may wear you down so that you are tempted to cave in and relax your standards. But hang in there.
>
> You and your spouse may find the going rough and begin to question if you really were made for each other. And you may see your neighbors call an end to their marriages, and everyone seems happier while the two of you still struggle. But hang in there.

You may be led to believe you are out of touch and old-fashioned because you believe what the Bible teaches about sexuality and sexual purity. But hang in there.

You may believe the polls that tell you the majority don't want to see a change in the laws that allow a doctor to end the life of a baby inside his mamma's belly, but at one time the majority wanted me to believe I was three-fifths human because I was black. But please hang in there.

You may think it doesn't matter who you vote for or what your congressman does because the system is corrupt — and Christians don't belong in politics anyway. But hang in there.

You may wonder why after trusting God all your life you lose your job, default on your mortgage, and have to work at McDonald's. But hang in there.

You may feel as if you're all alone, that no one else is willing to stand by your side when the going gets rough, and that even God is no longer listening to you. If so, you're in good company and you're in a good place. So hang in there.

Well before I was born, a German immigrant settled in Detroit. Like so many Europeans who came to America after the war, he was drawn by the promise of opportunity and freedom. Although a pharmacist in Germany, his English wasn't good enough for him to pass the exam to practice here, so he took a job in an auto plant. For almost forty years he worked in the same plant. He had started a Bible study with a small group of men. He asked them to contribute to a fund he was starting to provide scholarships to Africans who wanted to come to the United States to go to seminary. Over the years his fund helped dozens of Africans — including a tribal chief — receive an education that prepared them to go back to their country and teach others about Jesus. When his church needed a new building but couldn't afford to hire a construction company, he volunteered his spare time to help build the church. He taught a Sunday school class in his halting English for more than twenty years, and whenever he heard of a need among the church folk, he quietly found a way to meet it. When he took his family to a restaurant, he always gave the waitress a gospel tract along with his generous tip. He never missed an opportunity to vote in an election, and when any new law was proposed that he felt compromised his Christian values, he joined others to fight it.

Shortly after he retired from the auto plant, he was diagnosed with inoperable cancer. It was a fairly aggressive strain that took its toll on his strength and kept him in constant pain, but he continued to find ways to aim his mirror at the true light of the world. Eventually, however, he was placed under hospice care in his home. As the end of his life on earth became more likely, someone asked him how he managed to stay so upbeat, given the circumstances.

"When I lived in Germany, I used to love hiking in the

Harz mountains near my home," he began. "I would reach a particular peak and look out over the landscape, and it was like you could see forever. But when I looked down into the valley, I noticed something. It was so green and lush with farms, and it dawned on me. The valley is where everything grows."

You may be in a valley right now. But according to the Bible, at the proper time you will reap a harvest if you don't give up. Sometimes it rains in the valley, but the storms of life bring the Living Water that helps you grow in stature before God and man. Sometimes it's dark in the valley, but the light of the Son brightens your path and leads you to your new home.

Whatever you are facing today, whenever the burden you are carrying seems too much to bear, remember this: God loves you so much that he is shaping you into the image of his Son, Jesus. And his Spirit is right there with you, whether you're in the valley or on the mountaintop.

What could possibly be better than that?

"In *all things* God works for the good of those who love him, who have been called according to his purpose" (Romans 8:28, emphasis added).

Epilogue

A friend of mine, who knows a lot more about writing than I do, told me that when I finished this book, I should set it aside for a few weeks and then go back and read it. He said that getting some distance from the manuscript would give me a fresh set of eyes to review it and make sure I didn't leave anything out. Good advice, because as I read through these pages, it occurred to me that while true hope only comes from God through his free gift of salvation, he also uses others as his special agents of hope. In other words, all along the way in this journey with cancer, God has sent people into my life at just the right time to cheer me up, to pray for me, or just to sit beside me during a long night in the hospital. I won't attempt to name them because it would fill too many pages, and I'm sure I'd miss a few. But I mention this because you just might be one of those special agents God wants to use to bring hope to someone else.

You may not be going through a dark valley right now, but someone close to you may be. The Bible uses the image of the human body to describe the church, mostly to point to the different gifts of people in the church. But I also like to think of the body when it comes to pain: when one part of the body hurts, the whole body hurts along with it. The apostle Paul wrote, "Carry each other's burdens, and in this way you will fulfill the law of Christ" (Galatians 6:2).

Whenever I have to return to the hospital, I have found that it doesn't take much to cheer up somebody who's having a bad day. And it seems to spread quickly to others. I remember the time I had to go to the cancer clinic for an eight-hour treatment. I saw this couple and their teenaged son. The mom looked like death warmed over, and the two guys didn't look much better. When the nurse came to take the mom into her room, I introduced myself to the dad and asked if it would be OK if I dropped by her room later to encourage her. He seemed so relieved that *anyone* outside of their family cared at all. So a few hours later, I went into her room and said, "Isn't this cancer thing great!"

She gave me one of those looks that told me I wasn't exactly lifting her downtrodden spirit, but I kept going.

"I've had cancer now for seven years, and it's taught me so many great things about myself and God, and it's making me a better person. You're going to be just fine. God's going to take care of you."

By now her husband and son had entered the room and I detected a slight smile at the corner of the woman's lips. She started asking me questions, and I was making jokes, like I usually do, and every time my nurse walked by, I'd try to hide so I wouldn't have to go back to my room. Before I knew it, we were all laughing and carrying on as if we were lifelong friends.

All because I decided to do for her what many, many others had done for me.

One of the great things about hope is that you can share it. It's what we are called to do as Christians, but we should never think of it as an obligation or a duty. Whenever I take the time to try to cheer up someone who is going through a rough time, I end up feeling so much better myself.

Remember that little Sunday school chorus — "This little light of mine, I'm gonna let it shine"? There have been a few places in this book where I've described a pretty dark world, but only because I know how much light you can bring to it. Look around you — your family, your neighborhood, your schools, your workplace. I can guarantee that you won't have to look very far to find someone who needs the hope you've been given. You don't have to be a preacher like me, and you don't have to say all the right words. Sometimes just a hand on someone's shoulder is enough to communicate a message of hope. Whenever I go back to my cancer clinic, I know I can always find someone to touch — someone to lift up out of their sorrow.

What about you? Can you think of someone right now who needs to know that no matter how bad it looks, it can all be good? Is there someone in your life who could use an email message that simply states, "I'm thinking of you"? Thanks to a radio interview that was broadcast nationally, I have people from all over the country writing and calling to encourage me, and these little messages of encouragement always seem to come just when I need them.

I boldly asked you in chapter 1 to not feel sorry for me. And while I meant it, I don't want you to forget about me either. People who are seriously ill or going through very difficult times in their lives don't want to be ignored. They want to know that someone cares. Whenever you reach out to someone, you are reaching out with the hands of God. I saw a poster once that showed a poor urchin sitting in a filthy gutter. The caption read, "Sometimes you're the only Jesus I see."

As members of Christ's body, we have the amazing privilege of shining his light on a world that is hurting. We have been given the hope of eternal life in heaven as well as the hope of God's comforting presence on earth. When we let that hope transform us, everybody we touch wants some of it.

Your assignment in a hopeless world? Celebrate hope. Catch it. Share it.

READ. WRITE. REPEAT.

More products inspired by the
major motion picture letters to God

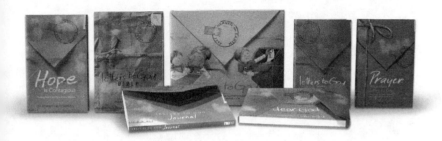

LETTERS TO GOD - THE NOVEL (ISBN: 9780310327653)
Now read the book behind the movie for a closer look at Tyler's story.

PRAYER: YOUR OWN LETTER TO GOD (ISBN: 9780310327639)
Strengthen your relationship with God. One prayer at a time.

LETTERS TO GOD - BIBLE (ISBN: 9780310949435)
This special Bible used in the movie features handwritten notes
and underlined verses to help you better understand Scripture.

LETTERS TO GOD - PICTURE BOOK (ISBN: 9780310720133)
Spark a child's imagination with this picture book based on the movie.

LETTERS TO GOD - JOURNAL (ISBN: 9780310720027)
Take your prayer to a new level by writing your own letters to God.

HOPE IS CONTAGIOUS (ISBN: 9780310327684)
Shows how to experience and spread hope in the face of every obstacle.

DEAR GOD (ISBN: 9780310327738)
Read Tyler's letters and get inspired to dig deeper into your faith.

For more information or to purchase these products
visit www.Zondervan.com or your local bookseller.

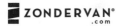

ZONDERVAN
.com

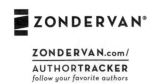